THE BOOK OF

MEDICAL EMERGENCIES

Your ready resource for first aid and emergency rescue

Dr Stuart Fischer

THIS IS A CARLTON BOOK

Text © Stuart Fischer

First published in the United States by Barricade Books Inc,
185 Bridge Plaza North Suite 308-A, Fort Lee, NJ 07024
www.barricadebooks.com

This edition published by
Carlton Books Limited 2006
20 Mortimer Street
London W1T 3JW

A CIP catalogue record for this book is available from the British Library

ISBN 1 84442 273 9

Printed and bound in Dubai

Dedication

This book is dedicated to Dr David Grob. I feel honoured to have been taught by him and to learn from his warm, caring and always inquisitive approach to the art and science of practising medicine.

– Dr Stuart Fischer

Contents

Acknowledgments

My most grateful thanks go to the following people, who contributed their time and expertise and helped make this book a reality. Dr Bertrand Agus (rheumatologist), Dr Sigmund Chessid (orthopaedic surgeon), Dr Avram Cooperman (surgeon), Dr Amy Glaser (paediatrician), Violet Kelly (the finest nurse I have ever worked with and an excellent teacher herself) and Susan Grisell, a prize-winning Impressionist artist who has stressed the relationship of man to nature, who contributed the illustrations.

We wish to thank and express our enormous gratitude to all of those who have helped and supported us in making this book a reality. Thanks especially to Rick Frishman, who brought us together and who has steadfastly been with us through this entire project.

Thanks also to Brian Waterbury, San Rafael, Martha Meador, Gay Lynn Duel, Margo Rohrbacher and Jeannie Huffman.

Introduction

At some point, you'll probably have to respond to a medical emergency. *HOW YOU RESPOND COULD SAVE YOUR LIFE OR SOMEONE ELSE'S.*

When a medical emergency arises, will you:

- Know what to do?
- Know what not to do?
- Know how to give and/or get successful treatment?
- Be able to help save someone's life?

In medical emergencies, knowledge is critical. You don't have to go to medical college or even learn complicated terms and procedures. However, you should – at the very least – get a basic understanding of medical emergencies that could affect you, your friends and loved ones. That is what this book provides.

Medical emergencies can range from superficial cuts and bruises to profound, life-threatening problems. Often, they're difficult to diagnose and distinguish. They affect not only patients, but families, friends and those who witness these often horrifying events.

The purpose of *The Book of Medical Emergencies* is to help non-medical people respond quickly and effectively to emergencies. To achieve this, it is written in the most clear, direct language, with a minimum of technical terms. All medical language has been clearly defined. This book has been designed to give readers easy access to vital information so they can act quickly and with confidence.

This book includes:

- Basic instructions on giving emergency care
- An explanation of how the emergency care system works
- Instructions (with illustrations) on how to perform CPR, take a pulse, stop bleeding wounds, support a fracture and tell whether the patient is breathing normally
- An index of symptoms to quickly diagnose emergencies
- Chapters devoted to each of the most common medical emergencies, which explain:
  1. What each emergency is
  2. How to recognize it
  3. What to do
  4. What not to do
  5. What treatment to expect at the hospital's accident and emergency unit
  6. Typical after-care
  7. Comments by a practising doctor

Keep a copy of this book in your home, workplace, car, boat and recreational vehicle. The information it contains could save a life!

Basic Principles of Emergency Care

1. Approach any emergency in a *calm* and *orderly* manner. When a patient is relaxed and confident, you increase the odds for a successful recovery. Diagnosis and treatment are easier and the patient is more likely to help – rather than hinder – medical personnel. Conversely, an alarmed patient can impede those who are trying to help. If you are the one giving first aid, don't panic or show your fears. If you are the one having the medical emergency, remain as calm as possible.

2. Be observant; take stock. Identify and assess the general nature of the problem. Is it an orthopaedic, surgical, medical or psychological emergency? Is the patient awake, responsive and comfortable? Is the patient unconscious? Can you feel a pulse? Has the patient stopped breathing (regardless of the reason why)? Are there any life-threatening injuries? Has the patient been removed from the source of danger?

3. If possible and if time permits, find out whether the patient has a pre-existing medical condition and which prescription medication(s) he/she is taking. However, do not put off calling 999 because you are busy conducting a lengthy search of the patient's medicine chest.

4. Call 999. When in doubt, call 999 as soon as possible. It makes absolutely no sense to delay, guess or take foolish chances when professional help is just a phone call away.

5. When you call 999, respond to the questions you are asked. The information you provide may be vital in saving the patient's life. Don't guess. If you don't know an answer, say so. The control officer will move on to the next question.

6. Ask the control officer what you can do until the emergency medical personnel arrive. Write down all instructions in the order in which they should be carried out. Emergency control officers are professionals who deal regularly with medical emergencies so make sure that you understand their instructions and follow them precisely. If you don't understand any instructions, ask for clarification.

7. Call friends and neighbours to assist or stay with you until emergency medical personnel arrive. Don't leave the patient unattended. If you don't feel up to the tasks at hand, get help.

8. When emergency medical personnel arrive, let them do their job. Follow their instructions and assist them if they ask for your help. Don't ask questions or get in their way when they are providing emergency care. Be patient. Let the experts do their work. You will have a chance to ask questions after they have stabilized the patient's condition.

9. Stay nearby. Be available to answer questions or to provide any assistance they request.

How Emergency Systems Work

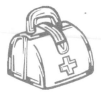

Emergency medical systems use a 'triage' or priority system, which operates both before patients reach the hospital and upon arrival. Basically, here's how it works.

1. When 999 calls are received, the control officer sends highly trained emergency medical personnel (ambulance and paramedic staff) to the scene. The control officer questions callers and sends emergency personnel to the most serious incidents first. The officer also relays all information that you provide to the emergency personnel, often while you are still on the phone.

2. Upon arrival at the scene, the emergency medical personnel evaluate the patient's condition. They may rely heavily on your observations. The medical personnel initiate treatment and decide whether and where to take the patient. When dealing with heart attacks, they may radio a doctor who will direct them to give oxygen, an Intravenous (IV) drip and morphine, heart drugs (e.g. glyceryl trinitrate) or other medication. A patient suffering from multiple, life-threatening injuries may be rushed to a special trauma centre rather than the accident and emergency unit of a general hospital.

3. Upon arrival at hospital, patients with the most serious conditions are seen first, their problems are diagnosed and treatments are started. Diagnostic testing usually includes obtaining the patient's history, a physical examination, X-rays, electrocardiogram (ECG) and blood tests. Some emergencies (hip fractures) may be immediately apparent, while

others (aortic aneurysms) may be more elusive. When you go to an emergency room, the first person you will talk to is a triage nurse, whose duty it is to prioritize your medical problem. Triage is a concept first formulated on the battlefield, where those individuals with the most severe treatable injuries needed to be attended to first. Because of the varied nature and enormous range of typical medical emergencies, your particular problem may not be dealt with immediately (cardiac and·trauma patients always have priority) and you may need to wait to see a doctor. Moreover, some emergencies need diagnostic tests to be performed (blood tests, X-rays) that will lengthen the time the patient will stay in the hospital. Many hospitals also have minor injuries (MI) units that can treat small wounds, such as cuts, grazes, minor burns and non-life-threatening bites and stings. The medical staff at the unit will assess whether an injury is serious enough to require transfer to the main hospital.

4. Many conditions may take hours to diagnose precisely. Specialists may be required. So be prepared to wait. Bring warm, comfortable clothing, reading material and lots of patience. You may find you receive the attention of a bewildering range of medical staff, in addition to doctors and nurses, including radiographers and medical technicians, consultants and even student nurses and doctors, who are sitting in on the examination as part of their training. However, all medical staff will try to put you at your ease and will be only too happy to explain anything that you are concerned about in order to allay any fears you may have.

When You Call 999

1. The first thing you hear will be, '999. Which service do you require?'

   - The 999 operator is a highly trained professional who knows the right questions to ask and is there to help.
   - Tell the operator if it is a medical emergency, a fire, a hazardous material spill, etc., if you know, and which of the emergency services you require. The options are fire, police, ambulance and – where appropriate – coastguard, mountain rescue and cave rescue. You will then be put through to the control officer of the service you require.
   - As briefly as possible, tell the control officer the victim's condition. For example, 'My husband isn't breathing', 'My son is bleeding profusely', 'He won't wake up.'
   - Briefly tell the control officer what happened. 'He just collapsed in the kitchen', 'He fell off a ladder', 'She overdosed.'
   - Get to the point. The more information the control officer gets quickly, the more it will help. While you are giving the information, the control officer may be relaying it straight to the emergency personnel.
   - Be calm and try not to panic. Your response could frighten the victim, which could worsen his/her condition and make it difficult for the control officer to get important information.

2. Know the correct address. Although the control officer will know the address where the call was placed, you will be asked to verify the address where the emergency personnel should go. This is necessary because you may be calling from a neighbour's house, from a public place or on a mobile phone.
   a. If you are calling from somewhere other than your home, know the address.
   b. If you are calling from a large public place, describe as precisely as possible where the victim is.
   c. If you are in a large store, a shopping centre or a place that has multiple entrances, ask somebody who works there which entrance is best for the emergency team to make for.
   d. If you are calling from a mobile phone, know where you are and where the emergency team should go.

3. Remain on the phone until the control officer tells you to hang up. If you hear a click or silence on the other end, don't hang up. Assume that the control officer placed you on hold while emergency help is dispatched. Expect the control officer to get back on the line to ask you additional questions.

4. Let the control officer take command. Control officers are trained to deal with panicked callers. Some distressed callers can waste valuable time by being long-winded, impatient, argumentative and even hostile. Keep calm, cool and focused. Trust the control officer and pay attention!

5. Be prepared to answer follow-up questions, such as 'What caused the fall?', 'Has this happened before?', 'How far did he fall?', 'Is he taking medication?' Once the emergency workers are on their way, the control officer may ask you for further information and relay your answers to the emergency personnel.

6. Follow the control officer's instructions. If she tells you to perform a procedure, she will explain exactly what you should do, step-by-step. She may tell you how to apply direct pressure to a wound, perform cardiopulmonary resuscitation (CPR) or clear a blockage with abdominal thrusts (Heimlich manoeuvre).

7. Many 999 centres have multilingual capabilities. Operators will find out what language you speak and instantly contact a translator who speaks your language and will join you in a three-way conversation.

Emergency numbers in the EU and the USA
The European Union emergency number 112 can also be accessed in the UK and should be used in all EU member states. In the USA call 911.

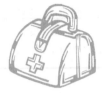

What Is an Emergency?

In this book we try to give guidance as to what constitutes an emergency and therefore when it is appropriate to phone 999. In many cases the situation will be clear cut. You should phone 999 if a person is having difficulty breathing, is unconscious, bleeding heavily, has received back, neck or head injuries, or has suffered serious tissue damage through chemical, electrical or fire burns. With respect to pregnant women who are having contractions, an emergency exists when there is inadequate time to safely transfer the patient to another facility before delivery or when the transfer might threaten the health of the mother or her unborn child.

However, there may be potentially serious or even life-threatening situations that are not as straightforward as this. Or perhaps you are concerned that a person's health or condition is deteriorating and you are unsure what to do. In this situation you have several options. You can phone your GP's surgery and ask to speak to your doctor, make an appointment or arrange a visit. Outside normal surgery times the same phone number will put you through to an after-hours medical service that can provide medical advice or arrange for a doctor to make a home visit.

Free health advice and information is also available 24 hours a day, seven days a week through the NHS Direct service – phone 0845 46 47 – a confidential helpline that you can use if you have concerns about your own health or the health of a family or friend. The service can also put you in touch with self-help or support organizations, if necessary. When you phone NHS Direct, your call will be answered by a highly trained operator who will ask you various questions in order to ascertain the exact nature of the problem. The operator will then suggest an appropriate course of action. In some cases you may be put through to a nurse, who can ask more detailed medical questions and may give self-help advice for you to follow. If the nurse thinks it is more appropriate, your details may be passed to your doctor or the after-hours service, who will contact you and may arrange a home visit. If the operator or nurse thinks the problem is serious he/she will contact the emergency services on your behalf and relay information to them directly.

Many cities and large towns in the UK now have a 'Walk-In Health Centre' or similar medical facility, usually attached to a major hospital, where you can seek medical advice and treatment without an appointment. When you enter the centre you will first speak to a nurse who will take your details and ask you about the problem. You will then need to wait until a nurse becomes available who can examine you and provide treatment or, if he or she thinks it is more serious, refer you to your GP, or the main hospital itself.

More information

You can also access information and advice on health and first aid via the Internet:

- For general health advice go to www.nhsdirect.nhs.uk
- For first aid information go to www.redcross.org.uk/firstaid

Medical Emergencies

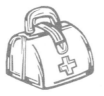

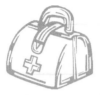

Abdominal Pain

What It Is

Although abdominal pain is often listed as the number one cause of accident and emergency (A&E) visits, the complex anatomy of the digestive tract can make it difficult to diagnose the precise cause of the pain. Abdominal pain may be due to one of more than 20 different illnesses or to injury (trauma). Pain may come from a ruptured or inflamed organ or from irritation or inflammation of the inner lining of the abdominal cavity (the peritoneum). The causes of abdominal pain can be grouped into four anatomical categories:

- Gastrointestinal: appendicitis, gallstones, intestinal obstruction, pancreatitis and diverticulitis.
- Genitourinary: kidney stones and urinary retention.
- Gynaecological: ectopic (tubal) pregnancy and pelvic inflammatory disease (PID).
- Vascular: ballooning of the aorta (aortic aneurysm), abdominal angina.

Some abdominal conditions pass quickly, while others are chronic. Abdominal pain may come on gradually or suddenly, be continuous or intermittent, and range from mild to excruciating. To complicate matters, it may be life-threatening or of minor significance and the cause can be unrelated to its apparent location ('referred pain' – for example, feeling right shoulder pain during gallstone attacks). Conditions such as gallstones, bleeding ulcers, appendicitis and kidney stones have several symptoms in common, so even mild and vague abdominal pain must be considered potentially significant.

Other causes of abdominal pain include small bowel obstruction (due to scarring from prior abdominal surgery), intestinal strangulation (a twisting of the intestines that cuts off the blood supply), pancreatitis (usually due to alcoholism or gallstones), diverticulitis (inflammation/infection of small pouches in the large intestine) and kidney disease (renal colic). Abdominal pain may also indicate cardiac disease since the lower portion of the heart shares nerve fibres with the upper gastrointestinal organs.

Gastrointestinal Bleeding

Bleeding may occur anywhere along the gastrointestinal tract; in the oesophagus, the stomach (peptic ulcers, erosive gastritis), small intestine (duodenal ulcer), large intestine (fragile blood vessels in the colon, diverticulitis or colon cancer) or the rectum (internal or external haemorrhoids). Virtually all patients with gastrointestinal bleeding will require medical attention (haemorrhoids can often be treated with over-the-counter creams and suppositories). The treatment will vary according to each patient's condition and the amount of blood loss.

What to Look for
- Paleness, pain, rigidity and severe tenderness over the entire abdomen may indicate **peritonitis, the most serious abdominal emergency**. Peritonitis results when an organ ruptures into the abdominal cavity, irritates the inner lining and shuts off all gastrointestinal functions. The abdominal muscles become tight and severely painful to touch.
- Nausea, vomiting, diarrhoea or unstable blood pressure (manifested by dizziness, severe fatigue or 'feeling cold').

- Watery diarrhoea, vomiting and abdominal cramps, but no localized abdominal pain, tenderness or signs of peritonitis (acute gastroenteritis caused, for example, by a virus or salmonella bacteria).
- Abdominal pain in an elderly patient with severe arteriosclerosis, hypertension, cold feet and leg cramps when walking may indicate an aortic aneurysm. This is a major medical emergency. Call 999 immediately.
- Abdominal pain, nausea and vomiting that are triggered by exertion and are relieved by rest (or glyceryl trinitrate) can indicate a heart problem. Call 999 immediately.
- Sudden onset of abdominal pain in children or the elderly can indicate appendicitis. The pain may develop anywhere in the abdominal area to begin with, but it will usually start around the belly button and then go on to localize in the lower right region after 24 hours.
- Rectal bleeding, black bowel movements or vomiting blood or 'coffee-grounds' material (gastrointestinal bleeding).

What to Do

- Call 999 immediately when abdominal pain lasts more than a few minutes and the patient feels faint or turns pale.
- Call 999 immediately if an elderly patient with severe arteriosclerosis, hypertension, cold feet and leg cramps has abdominal pain.
- Call 999 immediately if abdominal pain, nausea and vomiting occur with exertion and are relieved by rest or glyceryl trinitrate.
- Keep a patient who doesn't feel dizzy or look pale sitting down and leaning slightly forward.
- Keep the patient relaxed and comfortable.

What Not to Do

- Don't attempt to diagnose or treat anything but the most minor gastrointestinal symptoms (such as heartburn occurring after large, rich or spicy meals).
- Don't give a patient with potentially serious abdominal pain anything to eat or drink.
- Don't allow a patient to lie on his/her back, because vomiting may occur. Instead, turn the patient to one side.

Typical Treatment

The A&E staff will question the patient about the onset, nature, intensity, duration and apparent location of the pain. The patient's vital signs will be taken and may reveal low blood pressure and a rapid heart rate, which suggest loss of fluid (pancreatitis) or haemorrhage (perforated ulcers). Intravenous fluids are immediately given to stabilize the patient's circulation. Physical examination of the abdomen may reveal the root of the problem and/or the existence of peritonitis. Blood tests, X-rays and other imaging procedures (ultrasound, computed tomography – CT – scans, colonoscopy) may also be employed.

Laboratory and X-ray tests are required to diagnose pancreatitis, gallstone attacks and often appendicitis. All women of childbearing age will receive a pregnancy test to rule out ectopic pregnancy, which accounts for many surgical emergencies.

Pain medication cannot be given until the cause of the pain is determined because it might mask the manifestations of an illness (or even peritonitis). Before a treatment plan is set, the patient's condition will be confirmed and reconfirmed by:

1. Reviewing the history of the illness
2. Physically examining the patient
3. Analysing laboratory tests (blood, urine and X-ray)

Specific treatment will vary depending on the condition diagnosed. Treatments might include surgery for a ruptured spleen, intravenous fluids for kidney stones, antibiotics for diverticulitis, or all of the above for appendicitis.

The length of a hospital stay will depend on how quickly the patient is treated and whether complications develop. It may range from several hours for a mild intestinal virus to several weeks for repair of an aortic aneurysm.

For gastrointestinal bleeding, a tube may be placed through the patient's nose to wash out the stomach. Blood is an irritant and may be removed from the gastrointestinal tract. Internal bleeding may be treated during an endoscopy, the procedure performed to inspect the inner walls of the oesophagus, stomach and large intestine. After severe gastrointestinal bleeding, the initial blood tests may be misleadingly normal.

After-care

A patient with abdominal pain will be hospitalized unless his/her symptoms resolve completely in a few hours. Even a patient who doesn't require hospitalization should be re-evaluated within the next 24 hours.

The A&E staff will determine whether a surgical consultation is warranted. A patient with a ruptured aortic aneurysm or appendicitis complicated by peritonitis may be rushed to surgery within an hour.

Some episodes of abdominal pain are of brief duration and unknown origin. A patient diagnosed with 'nonspecific abdominal pain' will be ordered to see his/her GP within 24 hours or to return to A&E if the symptoms persist or worsen.

Acute appendicitis may resolve if faecal material blocking the entrance to the appendix is dislodged and passes through the intestine.

Surgery complicated by peritonitis may require hospitalization for a month or longer.

Doctor Says

To examine the abdomen, gently push down about 1cm (1/2in) and circle around the belly button. If the area feels as hard as wood and the patient is pale, suspect peritonitis and immediately call 999. Some facts: appendicitis is the number one cause of abdominal pain for patients under age 50; gallstones are the primary cause of abdominal pain for those over 50.

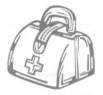

Appendicitis

What It Is

The appendix is a tiny, fingerlike pouch that sits at the end of the small intestine to the right of the belly button. Although it has no known function, it can cause serious emergencies, usually in children and adolescents. Most cases of appendicitis (and diverticulitis) occur when hardened fragments of faeces block the pocket's tiny opening and restrict the normal secretion of mucus into the intestine, causing the appendix to swell. Trapped bacteria flourish and attract cells from the immune system in nearby tissues. In worst-case situations, untreated swelling and infection can block the blood supply (causing gangrene) or rupture into the abdominal cavity (causing peritonitis), a life-threatening emergency.

High-risk groups include children, pregnant women and the elderly. Children under six have a high rate of perforation and peritonitis.

What to Look for

- WARNING: Whenever a child has abdominal pain, suspect acute appendicitis, no matter how slight, no matter what area seems to be affected. A running, playing or eating child is unlikely to have appendicitis. However, a child who has pain when coughing may have peritoneal irritation.
- Initial mild discomfort in the centre of the body around the belly button usually moving to the right lower abdomen over a four- to 48-hour period.
- Pain in any area of the abdomen or even in the lower back. The symptoms for acute appendicitis can resemble many other disorders. For example, the pain and

discomfort may be mild and resemble heartburn. Elderly patients (or those taking corticosteroids) may have more vague discomfort or no symptoms at all.
- Nausea, vomiting and loss of appetite.
- Mild fever – especially in young children.
- Discomfort and immobility.

What to Do
- Call 999 immediately.
- Keep the patient immobile. Unnecessary movement could cause the appendix to rupture and send bacteria into the abdomen. When in doubt, always err on the side of caution and call 999. The problem could quickly become serious and most GP surgeries lack the proper equipment to diagnose this emergency.

What Not to Do
- Don't give the patient medication, painkillers or other remedies. They could mask important symptoms.
- Don't touch or examine the patient. Touching could worsen the pain.

Typical Treatment
Diagnosis of acute appendicitis is based on the progressive development and migration of the patient's pain. Acute appendicitis may resolve if the faecal material that blocked the entrance to the appendix is dislodged and passes through the intestine.

The potential for serious complications makes exploratory surgery the best treatment. Furthermore, standard tests can be misleading. When peritonitis is suspected, the appendix will be surgically removed without waiting for test results.

As a result, surgery is often performed on patients even though as many as 20 per cent of them may not have appendicitis. When the diagnosis is less clear and the patient's condition seems less severe, ultrasound or computed tomography (CT) scans of the lower abdomen may be arranged. If they reveal an inflamed, enlarged appendix, the appendix will be surgically removed.

Uncomplicated appendicitis cases require only a few days' hospitalization. However, when an appendix ruptures and bacteria spread into the abdomen, surgery becomes more involved. In addition to removing the ruptured organ, the entire area must be cleansed to prevent the formation of adhesions (scarring) and abscesses.

A postoperative patient may remain on intravenous antibiotics for several days or weeks depending on the severity of the condition. The patient is not allowed to eat for several days after surgery because the gastrointestinal tract shuts off and food cannot be properly digested until normal operation resumes.

After-care

Appendicitis usually requires little after-care. When surgery is performed, one or two follow-up visits are needed to check on how the incision is healing.

A patient who is discharged from an accident and emergency (A&E) unit with an unclear but suspicious diagnosis should see a doctor within 12 to 24 hours. The patient should not take painkillers (including aspirin) or antibiotics unless authorized by a doctor.

Doctor Says

About 6 per cent of us have had our appendix removed. Do you still have yours? Originally, the appendix was probably a mini-storage area that functioned like one of a cow's three stomachs to help with the digestion of grass. However, as the human diet changed over millions of years of evolution, the appendix became unnecessary. Unnecessary or not, it can still cause problems and severe pain.

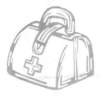

*Back Injuries**

What They Are

Essentially, the spinal column is a stack of small bones (called vertebrae) that surrounds and protects a network of nerves. The nerves connect the brain to a vast system of receptors, muscles and organs throughout the body. The vertebrae sit one on top of another, supported by muscles and separated by discs (softer, elastic cushions that help us bend and twist). An irritated or inflamed ligament, tendon, muscle or bone in the lower back can generate intense pain. About 85 per cent of the time, no definitive diagnosis or precise source of the back pain is found.

Some people are prone to back injuries because of inherent, inborn spinal weaknesses, but most injure their backs when they strain to lift heavy objects or lift objects in an awkward manner. These movements disrupt the spinal column's alignment and damage ligaments and tendons. Discs may slide out of position, compressing or irritating nerves; discs may also rupture and disc material may ooze out, compressing or irritating nerve roots. To prevent discs from slipping and causing further damage, the muscles in the area contract into a spasm. Although back spasms are painful, they prevent movements that could cause serious neurological damage.

Sciatica occurs when an injury to the lower spine irritates the nerve roots that form the sciatic nerve. This sends pain through the buttocks, down the back of the thigh,

---

* Cervical spine or neck injuries are discussed in a separate chapter called Neck Injuries.

and down the leg on one side of the body, often as far as the toes. A patient typically feels lower back pain, 'pins and needles' sensations or numbness in one foot. The patient may also limp or favour one leg and/or find it uncomfortable to sit or stand.

Spinal stenosis is a narrowing of the central spinal canal that is often mistaken for sciatica. As the cord compresses, it causes numbness in both legs that creates difficulty walking. Spinal stenosis is a degenerative condition that often accompanies osteoarthritis and is not due to physical injury. Sitting often helps to relieve the pain. Fractured vertebrae can cause the spinal column to partially collapse. Spinal fractures are painful and are usually caused by osteoporosis (a gradual process of bone loss more common in older women) injury, or cancer that has spread to the spinal column.

What to Look for

- Severe back pain, or 'pins and needles' (tingling and numbness of the arms or legs). Pain may intensify with physical movement.
- Shooting pain down the buttocks and leg (sciatica) or in the shoulder and arm.

What to Do

- Most patients with back pain don't need to call 999.
- However, you should call 999 if pain:
  - occurs suddenly
  - occurs immediately after strenuous physical exertion (or within 24 hours of it)
  - is triggered by a cough or sneeze
  - is excruciating

A doctor may not have the necessary medical equipment to assess the condition and may refer the patient to an orthopaedic surgeon or an A&E unit. Most patients with lower back pain can sit in a car long enough to get emergency treatment.

- Call 999 when any of the following neurological symptoms occur for the first time:
  - tingling ('pins and needles')
  - pain radiating down the leg
  - numbness
  - difficulty walking
  - loss of bladder control

What Not to Do

Don't move a patient who has sustained a back injury. Also, do not allow the patient to walk or move until healthcare professionals arrive. Movement can cause permanent neurological damage.

Typical Treatment

Since muscle spasms usually prevent disc slippage, most lower back pain does not involve nerve compression. Therefore, treatment focuses on the spasms. Oral muscle relaxants such as diazepam or methocarbamol are prescribed, as are anti-inflammatory medications including ibuprofen.

Although X-rays of the affected area are usually taken, they only reveal bone damage such as fractures. X-rays don't show damage to nerves, discs, ligaments and tendons or muscle spasms.

If nerve injury is suspected, a CT scan or magnetic resonance imaging (MRI) will be ordered to view the soft tissue between vertebrae. Patients will remain hospitalized only when emergency surgery is required.

After-care

Recovery and after-care depend on the severity of the condition and how quickly it was diagnosed and treated. Bed rest does not speed recovery from sciatica, but two or three days of bed rest on a firm mattress are still usually recommended.

Most patients are urged to resume their normal activities as soon as possible. They are given exercises to perform and instructions on proper lifting and bending techniques.

Chiropractors, osteopaths and acupuncturists can often relieve sudden back pain, but only if X-rays are negative and 'slipped' (prolapsed or herniated) discs are not suspected. Many patients with chronic low back pain benefit from physical and rehabilitative therapy.

Doctor Says

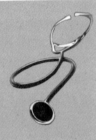

When a patient has 'pins and needles' sensations, call for emergency medical assistance immediately, especially if they were triggered by a cough or sneeze. Within two months of an injury, the condition of 90 to 95 per cent of all patients will improve, regardless of the type of treatment they receive.

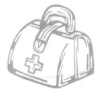

Bites and Stings

Human and Animal Bites

What They Are

Human, dog, cat and other animal bites account for 1 per cent of all A&E visits. Insect stings and injuries caused by poisonous creatures (rare in the UK) are discussed in this chapter. Injuries involving dangerous sea creatures (also rare in the UK) are discussed on page 131.

Human bites can transmit life-threatening infections because the human mouth contains anaerobic bacteria that flourish in the absence of oxygen. Unrecognized infections can turn fatal after 12 hours. Human bites occur almost exclusively on the hands or arms from intentional bites or from punches that contact the teeth. Herpes, hepatitis B and HIV viruses can also be transmitted through bites.

Dog, cat and other animal bites can puncture the skin, crush tissue and bones, cause infection and – rarely in the UK – transmit rabies. Although damage from most bites is superficial, serious injuries can occur that require immediate medical treatment. For example, a bite that just barely breaks the skin can still cause a serious infection. Infections emanate from bacteria in the animal's saliva. The likelihood of infection is influenced by the animal's size, the puncture's depth and the patient's age. Children and the elderly are most prone to infections.

Cat bites occur far less frequently than dog bites. But cat bites and cat scratches can cause more infections than dog bites. Cats' sharp and thin teeth can penetrate deeply, injuring tendons, nerves and blood vessels. These wounds are often hard to clean. Also, because cats frequently lick their claws, even minor scratches can easily become infected.

What to Look for

With the Animal

- The type of animal involved. Rabies is extremely rare in the UK, but a slight risk exists from smuggled pets. In the UK bats are potential rabies carriers, although the main risk is to licensed wildlife experts, the only people legally allowed to handle them. In foreign countries, any mammal is a potential rabies carrier, especially wild dogs and foxes, but also badgers and (in the USA) skunks and racoons.
- Foaming at the mouth, which indicates rabies.
- Whether the animal is wild, a stray or a household pet (in many countries pets are vaccinated).

With the Patient

- Bleeding.
- Open puncture wounds, cuts, scratches and scrapes.
- Swollen glands near the site of a cat scratch about one week after the scratch occurred.

What to Do

- Find out what kind of animal inflicted the injury. This may make a difference to the type of treatment required.
- Call 999 immediately.

- Find out if the animal was foaming at the mouth, wild or a stray.
- Check whether the wound is deep, open or continues to bleed.
- Stop the bleeding by applying gentle pressure to the wound with a clean cloth until the bleeding stops.
- Cleanse closed wounds with antiseptic soap or sterile water.
- Rush the patient to the nearest A&E unit.

Typical Treatment

Human bites are never stitched because some bacteria from the human mouth thrive in the absence of oxygen. Wounds are cleansed and irrigated with fluids, explored (if severe, in an operating room) and kept elevated. Intravenous antibiotics are given.

Dog, cat and other animal wounds are cleaned with antiseptic soap and sterile water. Large wounds will be stitched, but small wounds will usually be left open, irrigated and covered with sterile dressing. A patient will receive tetanus toxoid injections if he/she has not been immunized in the past five years. The patient will also be evaluated to see if minor surgery and/or antibiotics are needed. A cat bite victim is usually given antibiotics because cat bites are hard to clean.

When rabies is suspected, a patient is given immunoglobulin and booster vaccines.

After-care

Wounds usually close without the need for stitching. They should be examined every two to three days to monitor the healing process and check for infection.

A red streak leading away from the wound may indicate bacteria travelling through the tissues. This is a sign that intravenous antibiotics are needed.

Doctor Says

Each year, dogs are responsible for thousands of reported bites. Patients who were bitten by humans, however, are frequently too embarrassed to seek medical attention even though they may need it more than those attacked by animals. Make sure all human bite victims get prompt medical attention because they may not show signs of infection until 24 hours after they were injured.

Snake Bites

What They Are

Britain's only native poisonous snake is the European adder (or viper). This snake rarely bites humans and usually only attacks when it feels threatened. Its bite is rarely fatal but may pose a risk to children, the elderly and those with a serious medical condition or who suffer a severe hypersensitivity reaction (anaphylaxis). More exotic snakes are kept as pets, although usually only nonpoisonous species. The ownership of poisonous snakes is strictly controlled by law.

Britons are most likely to encounter dangerous snakes when abroad on adventure holidays, wildlife expeditions or when doing voluntary work in rural areas. Snake venom can damage the skin, heart and circulation and can affect the clotting system and blood pressure. Certain venoms can paralyse victims, impair their ability to breathe or cause internal haemorrhaging. However, even the most toxic snake venom usually takes hours or days to become life-threatening and modern medicine is highly effective, provided the patient receives prompt hospital treatment.

What to Look for

- Overall weakness.
- Pain, swelling and often burning pain around the wound.
- Pallor or cold, clammy skin (indicates internal haemorrhaging).
- Swelling, blisters or bruises around the wound.
- Numbness or 'pins and needles' feeling in the mouth, fingers and toes.
- Nausea, vomiting with subsequent chills and fever and sometimes blurred vision.
- Muscle paralysis.
- Difficulty breathing, swallowing or speaking.
- Seizures and/or muscle twitching.

What to Do

- Call 999 immediately.
- Check breathing and pulse. Be prepared to perform CPR.
- Keep the patient calm and motionless, because activity or fear can speed the spread of venom through the body.
- Remove rings and other jewellery, or loosen tight clothing.
- Gently wash wound area.
- Loosely place a constricting band (an article of clothing or an elastic bandage) between the wound and the heart to prevent the venom from entering the bloodstream. Keep the band in place until the patient receives professional medical treatment.

What Not to Do

- Don't move the patient. Movement can speed the spread of venom through the body.
- Do not let the patient eat or drink.
- Don't elevate injured limbs.

- Don't cut into the wound and try to suck out the venom. Cuts could injure tendons, nerves and blood vessels and may cause a serious infection.

Typical Treatment

Hospital treatment centres on cleansing wounds, administering antibiotics (whether the snake was poisonous or not), stabilizing the condition and, in severe cases, giving the patient antivenom to neutralize snake toxins. Adrenaline may be given to treat symptoms of anaphylaxis. Antivenom, including European viper antiserum, may be given intravenously. It is most effective when given within a few hours of the bite and can only be administered in a facility equipped to provide intensive care.

After-care

Snake bites may produce delayed reactions. Therefore, a victim must be observed for up to 12 hours after all acute problems have apparently resolved. In some cases the victim will be kept in hospital and monitored for at least two days. A doctor must re-examine the wound within 24 hours of discharge.

Doctor Says

It may be worthwhile to identify the type of snake involved because a patient's reaction and the treatment received may vary according to the type of snake that attacked. However, remember that time is of the essence – so don't let the identification of the snake interfere with or slow down a patient's treatment.

Insect Stings

What They Are

Stinging insects, such as bees, wasps and hornets, can cause major emergencies. A swarm attack can administer a potentially fatal dose of poison. An insect sting around the mouth may cause swelling that can block the airway. People who are allergic to insect stings may suffer a severe hypersensitivity reaction, known as anaphylaxis, which can be life-threatening. In some cases a sting may trigger an asthma attack.

When ticks bite, they burrow into their host's body to take and infect its blood. Ticks can transmit Lyme disease and other infections. Tick bites don't usually require emergency treatment, but call your GP if you experience any symptoms. You are most at risk of contracting Lyme disease in country parks, heaths and forested areas where wild deer, the tick's natural host, are found. Symptoms may include reddening at the site of the tick bite, fever, headache, fatigue, muscle pain and joint inflammation.

Bites by mosquitoes, horse flies, bedbugs, fleas and lice may transmit infectious diseases of varying levels of severity. Usually, they cause only unpleasant localized reactions and patients do not become hypersensitive to their bites.

In the UK it is rare to encounter deadly insects, spiders and scorpions. Some European spiders that can give a bite equivalent to a wasp sting are becoming native to Britain. Occasionally poisonous spiders and scorpions turn up in imported fruit, the backpacks of foreign travellers or as escaped pets. UK citizens are most at risk while abroad. Virtually all tropical and sub-tropical regions of the world have poisonous spiders and scorpions. Before travelling abroad, find out about potential dangers, how to avoid them and who to contact for emergency medical aid (see page 214). Biting flies such as mosquitoes and sand flies spread potentially fatal diseases, so always take preventive medication, if available, and seek advice on measures to avoid being bitten.

What to Look for

Insect Stings

- Redness, itching and swelling around the site, the face, neck, lips or tongue. Call 999 immediately.
- Itching, irritation, redness, flushing or rash (urticaria) over the whole body (signs of severe allergic reactions).
- Wheezing, coughing, hoarseness, difficulty breathing or speaking (may indicate swelling of the upper airways, a major medical emergency).
- Plummeting blood pressure and collapse (anaphylactic shock).

Tick Bites

- Ticks clinging to or burrowing in the skin and/or inflammation.

Foreign Spider Bites

- Cramping, muscle spasms.
- Fever, chills.
- Tightness in the chest and difficulty breathing.
- Dizziness, nausea, sweating or seizures.

Foreign Scorpion Stings

- Agitation, nausea or vomiting.
- Muscle spasms.
- Rapid pulse and shallow breathing.
- Blurred vision or uncoordinated eye movements.

What to Do

Insect Stings

- Call 999 immediately if the patient has difficulty breathing (or hoarseness) or was stung in or around the mouth. If swelling of the respiratory passages develops, the patient's breathing could quickly be impaired.
- Call 999 immediately if the patient has redness, itching or swelling around the site, the body, face, neck or tongue. The faster signs appear, the more severe the emergency.
- Remove the sting with a sharp blade or tweezers and wash the area with soap.
- Find out if the patient is allergic. Allergic patients usually carry a 'pen' that injects adrenaline. For less sensitive patients, place a thick paste of meat tenderizer and water directly on the wound to reduce pain, itching and swelling.
- Apply ice packs to the wound to slow the absorption of venom into the tissues.
- Give less sensitive patients an oral antihistamine (for example, acrivastine or cetirizine hydrochloride). Have a doctor examine the patient ASAP because delayed allergic reactions could occur within the next 24 hours.

Tick Bites

- Remove the tick with tweezers or a sterile needle.
- Gently pull the tick's entire body off by its head.
- Wash the wound and apply antiseptic.
- Consult a doctor as soon as possible to see if antibiotics would be appropriate.

Foreign Spider Bites

- Capture the spider, if safe to do so, or make a note of any identifying characteristics. However, don't take time away from attending to the patient.

- Seek medical aid immediately, as some spider bites can result in severe tissue damage.
- Place cold compresses on the bite.
- Move the patient's body so that the bite is lower than the heart.

Foreign Scorpion Stings
- Seek immediate medical aid. Scorpion stings can't be treated in the field.

What Not to Do
- Don't try to squeeze out an insect sting with your fingers.
- Don't squeeze a tick's body.

Typical Treatment

Insect Bites
A patient with swelling of the breathing passages will immediately receive intravenous adrenaline. Nasal oxygen, intravenous antihistamines and, on occasion, intravenous corticosteroids may be provided. An asthmatic patient will be treated with an inhaled bronchodilator. The patient will undergo close observation in the intensive care unit for several days. A patient who only suffered localized skin reactions may receive the same medications (adrenaline, antihistamines, corticosteroids) by injection or pills.

Tick Bites
Removal of the tick is the highest priority. If Lyme disease is common in the area or suspected, a patient may be given oral antibiotics such as tetracycline.

Foreign Spider Bites

In most cases, patients are given muscle relaxants such as diazepam. Antivenom will be used only in severe cases and usually provides relief in two to three hours.

Foreign Scorpion Stings

Intravenous fluids and medications may be given to prevent cardiac and neurological damage. Antivenom is not administered.

After-care

The key to controlling insect bites is avoidance: either stay indoors or keep well covered and use insect repellent. Spray sparingly with pesticides. A hypersensitive patient should carry an insect sting kit whenever he/she might be exposed to any stinging insects. Sting kits contain a 'pen' filled with adrenaline, which can prevent life-threatening allergic reactions. Adrenaline is also effective for patients with severe allergic reactions to food.

Doctor Says

On holiday one day, I witnessed a tourist being stung by a bee. Within minutes, his face and lips blew up like a red balloon. Luckily, we were able to get him to the accident and emergency unit of the nearby hospital within a few minutes, where medical staff were able to stabilize his condition.

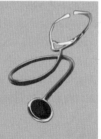

Breathing Disorders

What They Are

Shortness of breath is a symptom of a wide variety of conditions that affect the heart, lungs, circulation and metabolism. To operate, our bodies depend on a process called respiration, which delivers an uninterrupted supply of oxygen to our cells and removes carbon dioxide. If our oxygen intake drops, our bodies try to compensate by increasing the heart and breathing rate. A patient struggling for air may develop visibly abnormal intake patterns such as using his/her shoulders, ribcage or abdominal muscles to breathe.

Normally, we breathe 18 times each minute in a regular, calm pattern. Anything that hinders normal circulation and delivery of oxygen can significantly increase this rate.

What to Look for

- Rapid breathing, shortness of breath.
- Breathing through pursed lips – often related to emphysema, a disorder worsened by long-term cigarette smoking.
- Speaking one syllable at a time – indicating severe respiratory distress.
- Wheezing – a sign of asthma or fluid in the lungs.
- Blue lips, fingertips or tongue (cyanosis) – a sign of poor oxygen circulation.
- Inability to breathe while lying flat – if the patient is sitting up and struggling for air, it is usually due to severe congestive heart failure (also called pulmonary oedema or fluid in the lungs).
- Agitation or lethargy – signs of impaired delivery of oxygen to the brain.
- A choking noise (stridor) when the patient inhales.

What to Do

- Call 999 immediately if the lips, fingertips, or tongue turn blue and the chest wall doesn't seem to be moving. Perform CPR if needed (see page 192).
- After you call 999, don't leave the patient alone, because respiratory emergencies can worsen within seconds and you may need to perform CPR.
- Verify that the patient took prescribed medication as scheduled (for example, inhalants for asthma patients and oxygen for emphysema sufferers).
- Check the patient for signs of upper airway obstruction. Obstruction due to severe allergic reaction, certain childhood infections (such as croup) or from choking on food may be causing the shortness of breath.

What Not to Do

- Don't leave the patient alone.

Typical Treatment

Usually, the patient's history of respiratory problems and a physical examination will reveal the cause of his/her breathing problem. Other tests that may be ordered include arterial blood gas (to measure oxygen, carbon dioxide and pH), chest X-rays, electrocardiograms (ECGs), spirometry (to measure the patient's ability to expel air from the lungs) and haemoglobin levels (to check for anaemia).

Respiratory distress can also be attributable to heart problems (heart attacks, heart rhythm disturbances, congestive heart failure, angina), asthma, high blood pressure, blood clots in the lungs, allergic reactions, choking, carbon monoxide exposure and anxiety attacks. Rarer causes include collapsed lung, botulism and sickle cell disease (a genetic disorder mainly affecting those of Afro-Caribbean origin).

After-care

Further treatment will vary in accordance with the cause and the severity of the patient's specific respiratory emergency.

Doctor Says

'You have no idea how frightening it is to be short of breath,' one of my most brilliant professors, Dr Sidney Tessler, a lung specialist, would remind us. So take any sign of respiratory distress seriously and act quickly.

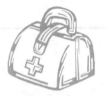

Burns

What They Are

Our skin keeps us warm, waterproof and free from external infections. More than 90 per cent of burns occur in the home and are relatively minor, but a small percentage may be life-threatening. Burns patients may suffer loss of fluid, reduction of body temperature and sepsis (bacteria multiplying in the bloodstream). The extent of any injury will depend on the duration, location, temperature and type of burn (that is, whether it is chemical, electrical or heat).

Burns disrupt body cell functions, hormonal balance, pH (acid–alkaline) balance and blood pressure. Inflammatory chemicals, such as histamine, are released that may extend the area of injury beyond the margins of the original burn.

Superficial burns will irritate exposed nerve endings and are usually painful. Deeper burns, including those that have been caused by scalding water, will kill cells and destroy arteries, veins and nerves. As a result of this, the patient may not feel any pain despite the damage that has been done.

Exposure to fire, smoke and ash particles may damage the upper airways, obstruct the flow of oxygen to the lungs and replace it with deadly carbon monoxide.

Burns are classified according to their depth: full thickness, partial thickness and superficial. Full-thickness burns go all the way to the bone; partial-thickness burns penetrate the skin, but do not reach the bone; and superficial burns injure only the outermost layer of skin.

What to Look for

- Redness, swelling and blistering of the affected skin.
- If a patient is coughing, wheezing or hoarse, call 999 immediately because the upper airways may be burned or filled with carbon monoxide.
- Seepage of tissue fluid. Seepage from extensive burns can cause a drop in blood pressure and impair circulation to the heart, brain and kidneys.

What to Do

- Separate the victim from the source of the burns.
- Call 999 immediately.
- Remove any affected articles of clothing.
- Check the patient's vital signs (see pages 190–91 and 207–8). If the patient has no pulse or is not breathing, immediately begin CPR (see page 192).
- Remove watches, belts, rings and jewellery that can retain heat and impair circulation to the arms and legs.
- Cool the area with cold water for at least ten minutes.
- Cover the burn in a clean dressing or plastic kitchen film to avoid infection.
- Check for damage to breathing passages, especially if smoke, gas, steam or fumes are present. Coughing up soot or blackened sputum can indicate breathing passage damage.

What Not to Do

- Don't apply ointments or cover the burn with butter, creams, lotions or other remedies.
- Don't cover the wound with bandages or any type of material that may stick to the fragile outer layers of skin.
- Don't apply ice to burns because it could cause additional tissue damage and may reduce body temperature too much.

Typical Treatment

If the patient is unconscious or his/her oxygen supply has been impaired, CPR may be required.

A patient burned on the mouth, tongue, nose or face may need intensive care treatment for upper airway scalding or fluid in the lungs (pulmonary oedema).

For deep or large burns, intravenous fluids will be needed to prevent circulatory collapse, brain damage and kidney failure.

If blood tests reveal carbon monoxide poisoning, high levels of oxygen will be given for several hours.

After the patient's blood pressure and respiratory status stabilize, dying skin may be removed surgically to prevent bacterial growth and scarring that could constrict the arms, legs or chest. Intravenous morphine is often prescribed for severe burns.

Burns specialists will determine what specific dressings, topical antibiotics or surgery are appropriate. A patient will be hospitalized for several days and longer if kidney or heart damage has been incurred.

After-care

A patient with minor burns usually does not require hospitalization. However, the patient must be re-examined within 24 hours by a doctor and specially trained nurses. A seriously injured patient will require more intensive follow-up after hospitalization. The healing process will be monitored and evaluated for three or four weeks. Scarring may be removed or improved by cosmetic surgery and skin grafts.

Doctor Says

Immediately assess the patient's breathing. If he/she is coughing up charcoal-like material or is not speaking normally, call 999 and be ready to perform CPR. The patient's upper airways could be inflamed, swollen and blocked, which could prevent breathing.

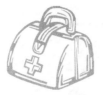

Choking

What It Is

There are two separate tubes or passages at the back of our mouths: the oesophagus, which carries food and liquids to the stomach, and the windpipe (trachea), the airway through which air enters and leaves the lungs. These two passages are not intended to be open at the same time so a small membrane, the epiglottis, seals the windpipe when we swallow.

When people simultaneously eat, drink, breathe, talk and don't adequately chew their food, the epiglottis may be overwhelmed. Food meant for the digestive tract may slip into the windpipe, where it gets trapped. Young children can inhale small objects such as beans, nuts, peanuts, erasers, pieces of toys, etc.

Coughing often dislodges obstructing objects, but victims can also hyperventilate and unintentionally force foreign bodies further down the windpipe. If the upper airway isn't completely blocked, victims may still be able to breathe. However, when the windpipe is totally obstructed, air cannot pass and victims can choke to death (the heart and brain cannot survive without oxygen for more than a few minutes). Mouth-to-mouth ventilation is ineffective since foreign bodies block the entry of air into the lungs.

What to Look for

- Coughing, gasping for air and/or clutching the throat.
- Fast and deep breathing.
- Change in the patient's voice (partial obstruction).

- Inability to talk (total obstruction).
- Wheezing (from trying to force air around the trapped object).
- Blue fingers, lips and face.
- Collapse, unconsciousness.

What to Do

Conscious Patient

- Call 999 immediately if he/she can talk, cough and breathe without assistance. Allow an alert patient with partial obstruction to try to clear the blockage on his/her own. Keep the patient erect, with his/her head leaning slightly forward.
- If the patient can't talk, breathe or cough, bend their head forward until it is lower than their chest and give five (5) blows between the shoulder blades, using the flat of the hand. For a child, place the patient over your knee and slap between the shoulder blades, using less force than for an adult. For an infant, place them along your forearm and use even less force.
- If this fails to clear the obstruction, perform five (5) abdominal thrusts (Heimlich manoeuvre). You should only perform this on adults and children over the age of one year old.

Abdominal Thrusts (Heimlich manoeuvre).

1. Stand directly behind the patient.

2. Wrap your arms around the patient's waist.

3. Clasp your hands above the navel under the ribcage so your thumb is pressing against the patient's abdomen. Be sure your hands are several inches below the lower tip of the patient's breastbone.

4. Pull inward and upward five (5) times in succession.

5. After each cycle of five (5) thrusts, gently sweep the patient's mouth with your finger to see if the object has popped out and can be removed.

6. Repeat the cycle of five (5) abdominal thrusts until the object dislodges, the person becomes unconscious or collapses, or emergency personnel arrive.

Unconscious Patient
- Call 999 immediately.
- If a patient inhaled vomit, place the victim on his/her stomach with the head as far down as possible. This should move the tongue forward and allow gastric contents to empty out of the mouth, not into the lungs. Then proceed as follows:

1. Turn the patient on his/her back and kneel alongside his/her hips facing the patient's head.

2. Deliver five (5) abdominal thrusts (Heimlich manoeuvre) by:
   a. Pressing the heels of your hands above the patient's navel, several inches under the ribcage. Be sure your hands are below the lower tip of the breastbone.
   b. Pushing inward and toward the shoulders five (5) times in succession.
   c. After each cycle, gently sweep the patient's mouth with your finger to see if the object has popped out and can be removed.
   d. Repeating the cycle of five (5) abdominal thrusts and checking the patient's mouth until the obstructing object is dislodged, the person becomes conscious, or emergency personnel arrive.

Choking Infants

- Place the infant on his/her back.
- Place two (2) fingers between the navel and ribcage and push downward and toward the shoulders several times.
- Check the child's mouth to see if the object popped out and can be removed. Proceed cautiously because it's easy to push objects back into the windpipe. Continue until help arrives.

If You Are Choking

- Stand facing the back of a chair or over a railing.
- Place your fist between your navel and ribcage.
- Lean downward quickly into the chair or railing so that your fist presses into the abdomen and upward towards the shoulders.
- Repeat until you feel the object pop out, until you can breathe normally or until help arrives.

What Not to Do

- Don't do anything other than call 999 if a patient is talking, coughing and breathing normally.
- Don't try to remove partial obstructions. You could force an unstable blockage further down and create a total obstruction.

Typical Treatment

Ambulance/paramedic personnel will try to dislodge the foreign body and will give the patient intravenous fluids and oxygen.

A tracheotomy (puncturing of the front of the throat to allow air to enter the lungs) may be required if an object is still lodged in the upper airway.

A seriously impaired patient will be hospitalized for a day or two to insure that he/she hasn't suffered lung damage or pneumonia. After X-rays are taken, a pulmonary (lung) specialist may inspect the upper airways and lungs with a special fibre-optic camera.

After-care

After an obstruction has been removed, the patient should sit quietly for a few minutes. Further care isn't usually required because momentary choking seldom causes significant cardiovascular or neurological damage. The patient should see a doctor immediately after a choking episode. Rib fractures and liver damage are rare, but possible, side effects of using abdominal thrusts (Heimlich manoeuvre).

Doctor Says

Choking can occur anywhere: at home, at work, in schools and colleges, in restaurants and at all social occasions. The St John Ambulance, the St Andrew's Ambulance Association and the British Red Cross all offer courses on first aid, including lessons on how to assist choking patients. You are strongly urged to attend!

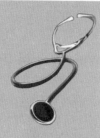

Cold Exposure

(Hypothermia)

What It Is

When our body is cold, we reflexively shiver to increase our blood flow, which delivers heat to our muscles. When our body temperature falls below 34.5°C (95°F), hypothermia occurs. In response, our respiratory, heart and brain functions slow dramatically in order to keep us alive. In effect, our vital organs go into hibernation, so hypothermia victims can survive for hours under frigid conditions.

Hypothermia is usually caused by exposure to freezing weather. It can also result from lengthy surgery (patients lose warmth in cold operating rooms), malnutrition, severe burns and dehydration. Loss of tissue fluid or blood, which normally spread heat through the body, can dangerously lower body temperature. Blood-borne infections, major injury that entails excessive bleeding and conditions that cause extremely low blood pressure also impair the delivery of heat to our tissues.

What to Look for

- Blue lips.
- Shivering.
- Unresponsiveness, confusion or disorientation.

What to Do

- Call 999 at once, *even if the patient seems dead*, has blue lips, isn't breathing or has no pulse. (Hypothermia victims can often be revived if they are transported immediately to an intensive care facility.)
- After notifying 999, begin CPR (see page 192).
- For an awake and responsive patient, check breathing and pulse every few minutes.
- Before the ambulance arrives, move the victim from the cold area, if possible.
- Replace wet clothing with dry, warm blankets, sheets or similar coverings.

What Not to Do

- Don't feed the patient because hypothermia usually shuts off stomach, intestinal and kidney functions. The patient could become nauseous and, if lying on his/her back, could choke on vomit.

Typical Treatment

Hypothermia, even when severe, is often reversible. The patient will be warmed with special blankets, heat lamps, heated oxygen and warm intravenous and gastrointestinal fluids. As the body temperature rises, the patient will be monitored for infection, kidney and liver failure, muscle destruction, heart rhythm disturbances and blood chemistry disorders.

It may take several days after the patient begins circulating the usual quota of warm blood for the kidney, liver and general metabolic functions to return to normal. In extreme cases, haemodialysis may be required. Haemodialysis involves placing catheters in the patient's abdomen to remove accumulated metabolic waste and restore the pH (acid–alkaline) balance. Recovery usually takes several days but may last several weeks for a patient with multi-system involvement and complications.

After-care

The patient should be re-examined by his/her GP or specialist within a few days of discharge from the hospital. Thereafter, recovery should be monitored with periodic blood tests and ECGs. A patient who was in critical condition usually requires several weeks of outpatient treatment.

Doctor Says

Usually, we picture stranded mountain climbers, skiers or boating-accident patients as the typical hypothermia victims. However, hypothermia more commonly strikes the elderly, rough sleepers, the intoxicated or the mentally ill who are found shivering or comatose on freezing streets. Often, these patients have wet or inadequate clothing. Alcohol, drugs or medication may have depleted their body heat or slowed their metabolism.

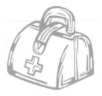

Cuts and Bruises

What They Are

The skin is the body's main protective surface. Cuts (lacerations) and scrapes (abrasions) provide openings through which infections can enter the body and precious bodily fluids can seep out. These injuries primarily involve the hands, face and scalp.

Bruises are superficial injuries of the blood vessels in the outermost skin layers. They do not provide an entry to deeper tissues and do not require antibiotics or stitches. Bruises that form small collections of blood under the skin (haematomas) usually disappear in a week or two.

Millions of wounds are treated every year in the UK, accounting for up to 10 per cent of all accident and emergency visits. When we are cut and bruised and also suffer major traumas, such as fractures or head damage, the potentially more serious injuries are examined and treated first.

Patients with diabetes, poor circulation or suppressed immune systems (for example, those taking corticosteroids) are more prone to skin infections. Infections are also more likely in injuries to the hands and feet.

Contaminated minor skin breaks can result in abscesses or cellulitis – dangerous bacterial growth in the deeper tissue layers.

Cuts and bruises may be signs of other medical conditions: sudden collapse due to heart problems, alcoholism, blackouts, epilepsy and even child abuse. These conditions may require greater attention than the cuts or bruises themselves.

What to Look for

- Breaks in the skin.
- Bleeding.
- Bacterial contamination. Find out what caused the injury, because dirty objects can cause infection.
- Foreign objects in the wound (glass fragments, thorns or splinters).
- How much time passed since the injury. Wounds should be examined as quickly as possible (within six hours) to prevent infection and promote healing.
- Infection: redness (including red streaks leading away from wounds), swelling, skin warmth, fever, pus and pain.

What to Do

- For cuts with little or slight bleeding, immediately place a sterile gauze pad or large bandage over the wound to stop the bleeding and prevent bacterial contamination.
- Remove all clothing, rings and jewellery from the affected area.
- When blood is flowing from a wound, gently place direct pressure over the wound. Elevate cut arms or hands as high as possible when transporting the patient to the hospital. Act promptly. Open wounds can become seriously infected within six to 12 hours and sealing or bandaging them may inadvertently cause rapid bacterial growth. Surgery can't be performed on infected areas; these must be initially treated with antibiotics and surgery delayed until the healing process has started.
- Puncture wounds rarely need surgical closure, but can easily become infected.

What Not to Do

- Don't apply hydrogen peroxide, iodine or any antibiotic creams or lotions to lacerations. They could enter the bloodstream and delay healing by injuring or over-moisturizing the area.

- Don't attempt to treat infections; leave it to trained medical staff.
- Don't apply tourniquets, because they can block the blood supply to the injured area.

Typical Treatment

After removing protective coverings, the extent of the injury will be determined. Minor, uninfected lacerations a few hours old will be cleansed and stitched, stapled or taped. A local anaesthetic may be injected first to numb the injured area. If nerves, tendons, bones or blood vessels were injured, more extensive surgical treatment will be required.

Lacerations more than 12 hours old usually won't be stitched because they are presumed to be infected. X-rays may be needed if foreign bodies such as glass, metal or gravel entered the lacerated area. Instead of stitching, the wound will be examined and cleansed with sterile water. Dead skin – fragments that have lost their blood supply – will be removed and wounds will be allowed to heal without surgery. Patients will be required to take antibiotics for at least a week. This is called secondary closure. A patient who hasn't received tetanus toxoid vaccinations in five to ten years will get booster shots. Wounds may be covered with a protective ointment, and dressed with gauze and bandages. Follow-up appointments may be scheduled for wound inspection and care.

After-care

Wound areas may be gently cleaned 24 hours after being stitched, but avoid bathing and soaking. Lacerations should be checked within 36 hours for possible infection and to monitor the healing process. At that time, the wound should be re-dressed.

Stitches should be checked after four days and, if no complications occur, they will be removed in seven to ten days. Stitched wounds that are healing should be inspected frequently during the next two to three weeks until they are completely mended. Most lacerations heal within three to four weeks.

Doctor Says

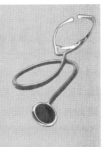

Get cuts and bruises examined promptly. When injuries are treated in the first six hours, the risk of infection decreases and the odds of successful healing increase. The signs of infections usually appear in the first four days, so be on guard. If the wound aches, burns, becomes inflamed or develops pus, get immediate treatment.

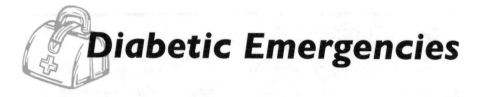# Diabetic Emergencies

What They Are
Diabetes is classified according to one of two categories:

Type 1 diabetes, which is rare but severe, is the permanent absence of insulin (the hormone that transports sugar into cells and so helps store energy). Instead of entering muscle and liver cells, sugar is released into the bloodstream. The onset of a type 1 diabetic emergency is often sudden and dramatic. A patient who was well one minute is suddenly in an intensive care unit fighting for his/her life the next.

Type 2 diabetes accounts for 95 per cent of all diabetic cases. It occurs when the pancreas does not put out sufficient insulin or the insulin it produces is ineffective ('insulin resistance'). Risk factors include obesity, inactivity and a genetic predisposition to the illness itself. A patient may not develop symptoms until the disease has caused major damage.

If uncontrolled, both forms of diabetes can cause a damaging rise of sugar in the bloodstream. Normal blood glucose ranges from 80 to 110mm per 100cc of blood (except when we eat). Emergencies usually occur when it dips below 60mg (if too much medication is taken) or soars above 400.

Infection, stress, pregnancy, severe burns, trauma and overeating can also elevate a diabetic's glucose. A patient can get 'insulin reactions' if he/she doesn't eat enough carbohydrate (starch or sugar) after taking prescribed diabetic medications. Excessive amounts of sugar enter the tissues, leaving too little for the brain to function effectively.

Cardiovascular diseases, such as heart attacks, angina pectoris and strokes, are more prevalent among diabetics. Diabetes may also incur organ-specific emergencies, including retinal detachment, kidney failure and leg ulcers.

What to Look for

- Excessive drinking of water, excessive urination and fatigue.
- Check for a diabetic emergency bracelet, which many diabetics wear.
- The inability to walk or move (may indicate low glucose in patients who have taken too much medication).
- Severe dehydration in frail, elderly diabetics (may indicate very high glucose).
- Confusion, dizziness or weakness may indicate either high or low glucose ('insulin reaction').
- Breath having a fruity scent, like apricot jam. Immediately call 999 because it may indicate diabetic ketoacidosis, an emergency where the lack of insulin is so severe and glucose so high, that fat molecules are released into the blood to supply energy to the cells.
- Rapid breathing, nausea, vomiting and abdominal pain (diabetic ketoacidosis).

What to Do

- If the patient appears nearly comatose (due to an 'insulin reaction' or overmedication) or seems to be slipping into a coma, give fruit juice, sugary drink or milk as soon as possible. If glucose is not restored within minutes, brain damage may occur.
- If the patient drinks and/or urinates excessively, call 999 or your doctor because his/her glucose may be elevated and dehydration or ketoacidosis could develop.

What Not to Do

- Don't confuse a diabetic emergency with intoxication. Always check to see if the patient has a diabetic bracelet.
- Don't minimize a diabetic's chest pain. A diabetic may develop serious heart problems with minimal or no symptoms.

Typical Treatment

Paramedics usually administer concentrated glucose intravenously for severely low sugar due to overmedication. An unresponsive, nearly comatose patient will improve within minutes and further treatment may not be needed.

A patient with extremely high glucose (over 400) will be hospitalized and given intravenous fluids and insulin injections to treat dehydration, lower blood sugar and correct blood chemistry imbalances. A patient with ketoacidosis will be monitored in the intensive care unit for several days and hourly blood tests may be required.

A type 2 diabetic with less severe complications will be hospitalized for several days to adjust his/her medication regimen and diet.

After-care

The patient should see his/her doctor for blood tests a week or two after being discharged from the hospital. Blood tests may identify problems with the patient's diet, medication regimen and other contributing factors such as infections.

Doctor Says

In Latin *diabetes mellitus* means 'sweet flow of water' because doctors in ancient Rome diagnosed diabetic emergencies by tasting patients' urine. Sweet-tasting urine indicated a metabolic crisis. Diabetes has grown to epidemic proportions in the West and millions more are expected to develop it in the next few years. Diabetics know how to check their sugar levels. Do you? If a diabetic is near and dear to you, learn to check his/her sugar levels. You could save a life.

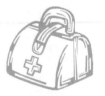

Diarrhoea

What It Is

Patients with diarrhoea have watery, loose, unformed stools or a dramatic increase in the number of their daily bowel movements. Severe diarrhoea can become a medical emergency if it causes dehydration, low blood pressure and electrolyte imbalances (particularly of potassium) that can damage vital organs.

Diarrhoea can be brought on by a wide variety of infectious agents including viruses (particularly in infants), bacteria (salmonella, shigella) and protozoa (amoebas, giardia). It can also be due to severe gastrointestinal illnesses (ulcerative colitis, Crohn's disease), stress ('irritable bowel syndrome') or the side effect of medical treatments (radiation therapy for cancer) or medications (antibiotics, chemotherapy).

Food poisoning from eating contaminated food, such as meat (especially chicken), fish, shellfish or egg products, is another common cause of diarrhoea. Symptoms usually appear within eight hours of intake, but they may not begin until several days later.

What to Look for

- Watery, loose, unformed stools (especially if lasting more than three days).
- Dramatic increase in the number of bowel movements.
- Nausea.
- Vomiting.
- Fever.
- Abdominal cramping.

- Inability to stand or unsteadiness.
- Light-headedness, faintness or dizziness.
- Excessive wind.
- Bloating or abdominal swelling.
- Abdominal pain.

What to Do

- Call 999 when patients complain of severe muscle cramps or cannot stand.
- If the patient feels faint, light-headed, dizzy or unsteady on his/her feet, call the doctor at once. The doctor may call an ambulance or direct you to call one.

What Not to Do

Don't administer over-the-counter antidiarrhoeal medications when patients have severe diarrhoea or cramps. Only doctors should direct their use. In infectious diarrhoea, the body is trying to rid itself of offending bacteria and toxins. So stopping the diarrhoea will keep toxins and bacteria in the gut, where they can spread and overwhelm the body's defences. Inappropriately administering medication could actually prolong the duration and severity of the patient's diarrhoea.

Typical Treatment

Patients with minimal symptoms do not usually require treatment. However, the elderly may incur unrelated cardiovascular complications if fluid loss isn't corrected. Therefore, hospital treatment will be needed, consisting of identifying the cause of diarrhoea and intravenous fluids, antibiotics, potassium and/or antidiarrhoeal medications.

A patient showing no symptoms after eight to 12 hours of A&E observation is usually discharged, which is the typical scenario with food poisoning. When a patient doesn't improve or has very low blood pressure, hospital admission will be necessary. The patient's blood will be tested to check the severity of the infection (for high white blood cell count) and potassium loss. Stool samples will also be analysed for blood, which may indicate severe gastroenteritis or other serious diseases (ulcerative colitis or colon cancer). Melaena – foul-smelling, black tarry stools – is usually due to a bleeding ulcer.

After-care

In most cases of infectious diarrhoea, after-care is rarely needed and a patient is seldom hospitalized for more than a few days. Patients with underlying diseases that caused their diarrhoea should undergo diagnostic tests (endoscopy of the colon or upper GI tract) and specific treatment for those disorders before their condition can be controlled.

Doctor Says

Don't treat the early stages of diarrhoea with over-the-counter medications – you may make it worse. If diarrhoea strikes while travelling, drink fluids to balance fluid loss and rest in bed until the crisis passes, usually in six to eight hours. Try to identify and avoid the offending food. In severe cases, make up an oral rehydration solution to replace lost salts and fluid. Dissolve one level teaspoon of table salt and eight level teaspoons of table sugar in 1 litre (1¾ pints) of cooled boiled water and sip every five or ten minutes.

Drowning

What It Is

Inhaling water rather than air can cause unconsciousness or death from lack of oxygen (asphyxiation). When the lungs fill with water, normal chest expansion is restricted and circulating oxygen decreases. This makes the blood more acidic, causing brain damage.

Drowning is often preventable. Victims are often healthy children who cannot swim, but about one third of all drowning cases involves swimmers who are overwhelmed by cold or dangerous waters, intoxicated by drugs or alcohol, or suffer sudden heart attacks. Usually, the first rescuers are not medical personnel (so it could be you!).

What to Look for

- Check if the patient is breathing.
- If the patient is not breathing, check for a pulse in the neck (see page 190).

What to Do

- Remove the patient from the water ASAP! Trained personnel, such as lifeguards or paramedics, may begin treatment while the patient is still in the water.
- Place the patient on his/her back and tilt his/her head slightly back. If the patient has no pulse, begin CPR (see page 192). The need for CPR is more urgent if the patient was under water for more than 30 seconds.
- Call 999 to assist in CPR, provide oxygen equipment and administer necessary medication.

- If the patient has a pulse, immediately start mouth-to-mouth (or mouth-to-nose) ventilation, one breath per three to four seconds (see the directions for mouth-to-mouth ventilation on page 193). Mouth-to-mouth breathing may stimulate the victim's respiratory centre and bring immediate improvement.
- Check continually to see if the patient is reviving or breathing on his/her own.

What Not to Do
- Don't try to squeeze water from a patient's lungs by applying abdominal or chest pressure. The patient may have swallowed large amounts of water that could be forced from the stomach into respiratory passageways, worsening his/her condition.
- Don't attempt abdominal thrusts (Heimlich manoeuvre). They do not help drowning victims and will impede CPR.

Typical Treatment

Oxygen will be provided as soon as possible and a patient in serious condition will be put on mechanical ventilation. Inhaling large quantities of water can damage lung tissue and the fluid overload can impair the patient's circulation.

Specialized blood tests (arterial blood gases) will measure how much oxygen and carbon dioxide the patient is circulating as well as his/her blood pH (acid–alkaline) status. Imbalances will be corrected during continuous intensive care monitoring.

A patient rescued from icy or freezing cold water may require treatment for hypothermia (see Cold Exposure/Hypothermia on page 63).

Although chest X-rays can diagnose pneumonia or lung damage, they will not show whether the patient's oxygen circulation is adequate or if all water has been removed.

After-care

A patient with balanced arterial blood gases is usually discharged within one to two days. However, a patient who suffered lung, heart or brain damage requires frequent follow-up. Cardiovascular and respiratory complications (heart attack, pneumonia or arrhythmia) may occur at any time, so intensive care must continue for several days until the patient is out of danger.

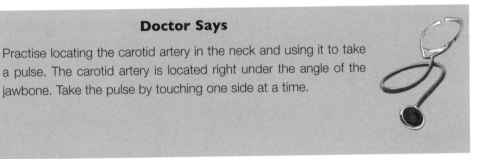

Doctor Says

Practise locating the carotid artery in the neck and using it to take a pulse. The carotid artery is located right under the angle of the jawbone. Take the pulse by touching one side at a time.

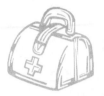

Electrical Injuries

What They Are

When our skin's surface is struck by more than 600 volts of electricity we die. The voltage can enter the body, penetrate deeply and kill tissue in its path. Although bones can withstand high temperatures, adjacent muscles, nerves and blood vessels can be destroyed by strong electrical charges. Patients with deep tissue damage often exhibit minimal external signs of injury.

The skin's resistance to electricity is lowered by water and even sweating. As a result, over half the deaths from electrical injuries are caused by low voltage jolts, such as those caused when electrical appliances (radios, hairdryers) fall into the bath.

High-voltage injuries, especially those received from lightning, can cause heart damage including rhythm disturbances (usually temporary), death of cardiac muscle and even cardiopulmonary arrest. When struck by high voltage, the body may shake with a single, powerful muscle spasm. Renal failure can occur when fragmented muscle cells block the small tubules of the kidneys.

Direct electrical damage to internal organs is rare because the current is usually spread over the large surfaces of the chest and stomach. In contrast, arm and leg injuries can be severe because there is less surface area to absorb the jolt. Patients can also be seriously injured when electricity ignites their clothing.

Most damage occurs immediately. However, delayed complications are possible, as in subsequent blood clots that block the blood supply to a hand or foot.

What to Look for
- Check the patient's pulse (see page 190) and breathing rate. Start CPR if the patient is not breathing or his/her heart is not beating (see page 192).
- Check for burns (remove clothing if necessary). The patient's internal injuries may be much worse than the visible burns you see on the surface.
- Seizures, loss of consciousness, agitation.

What to Do
- Identify, isolate and shut off the source of electrical current (if safe to do so).
- Call 999, even if the patient seems to have sustained only minor electrical injuries.
- Begin CPR (see page 192) if necessary.
- Cool the burn with plenty of cold water (if the electrical current is shut off).
- Cover with a clean dressing or plastic kitchen film until emergency personnel arrive.

What Not to Do
- Don't apply iodine, creams or antiseptics since they could be absorbed into the bloodstream.
- Don't allow the patient to move on his/her own. There may be deep tissue damage to the muscles and/or nerves.

Typical Treatment
A patient exposed to high-voltage electricity will be hospitalized and will receive continuous cardiac monitoring for several days. Those who were struck with lower voltage and experienced chest pain, pulse irregularities, amnesia, disorientation or agitation will also be given inpatient monitoring.

Heart damage and heart rhythm disturbances are the most serious concerns. A patient with these problems may require defibrillation and intravenous medication (lidocaine, beta-blockers). When the patient's cardiac condition has stabilized, the injured area will be examined to make sure that muscle and nerves adjacent to bones were not damaged. Intravenous fluids will be administered if the burned tissue sustained substantial fluid loss. Physical examination and Doppler ultrasound can determine the extent of circulatory damage.

Wounds will be cleansed with sterile fluids and burn creams that are only available by prescription. Since dead tissue is a potential source of infection, it may be surgically removed. If tissue swelling impairs circulation, fluid will be removed surgically, usually under sterile operating-room conditions. Amputation may be the only alternative if blood flow isn't restored after 24 to 48 hours of intensive effort.

The extent of injuries and recovery depends on factors such as the source of electricity, duration of exposure, amount of voltage, the anatomical path taken and the type of current involved (AC inflicts more severe damage than DC). A patient with fluid imbalance, infection or renal failure will require longer hospitalization.

After-care

Wounds will need to be re-examined every few days, preferably in a specialized burns unit. Examination will also take place in order to assess how musculoskeletal and nerve injuries are healing.

Doctor Says

Over 10 per cent of deaths from burns are due to electrical injuries. Most of us have received mild jolts from touching improperly wired objects. Fortunately, our reflex to withdraw from painful stimuli usually prevents serious consequences.

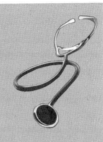

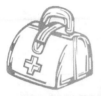

Eye Injuries

What They Are

Most common eye injuries result from foreign objects entering and irritating the surface of the eye. Dust, sand, soil or eyelashes usually cause minor irritation, while metal, plastic or glass fragments can create serious damage. Even contact lenses can scratch the cornea – the clear membrane that protects the pupil and lens. Scratches can be extremely painful, and pain and irritation can often linger long after the object is removed.

As most people age, gradual changes in their eyesight occur such as near-sightedness, far-sightedness, astigmatism and ageing eyes. Usually, they experience blurred vision that can be corrected by glasses. Cloudy vision can also be attributable to cataracts (whitening of the lens at the front of the eye) and glaucoma (increasing pressure inside the eyeball that produces haloes around lights).

Sudden loss of vision is usually caused by diseases of the retina (the thin layer of receptor cells at the back of the eyeball), diseases of the uveal tract (the organs that bathe and defend the inner eye) or impaired circulation and oxygenation of visual pathway nerves. When retinal receptors lose their blood supply, they quickly die and cannot be replaced. Since eyesight depends heavily on normal blood circulation, illnesses that constrict or block arteries can cause sudden loss of vision. Strokes involving the retina, optic nerve or the brain's visual processing centre can also cause irreversible damage. Risk factors for such strokes include hypertension, diabetes, high cholesterol and atrial fibrillation, which can cause dangerous blood clots.

When patients see 'flashing lights' or suddenly lose vision as if a curtain was raised before them, they usually have retinal detachment (the retina peeling off the back of the eye). Retinal detachment is often caused by uncontrolled diabetes and is a major cause of blindness. It can also be caused by injury to the head or eye.

Less threatening eye emergencies include conjunctivitis (generalized redness of one or both eyes), sub-conjunctival haemorrhages (small, benign collections of blood that do not cover the pupil) and styes (infections of the oil gland at the root of an eyelash).

Blows to the face may break bones that support the eyeball and cause it to droop. Patients who cannot look upward may have 'blowout' fractures and must be immediately examined, X-rayed and CT-scanned, otherwise their eye movements could be permanently damaged.

Bell's palsy, a drooping or paralysis of one side of the face, is caused by viral infections that affect the nerve that controls some eye movements. Patients may be unable to blink one set of eyelids. Bell's palsy is not a stroke and usually resolves on its own after about six weeks. However, Bell's palsy patients should be examined by a neurologist as a precaution.

Temporal arteritis produces sudden loss of vision in one eye accompanied by a throbbing headache on the same side. If immediate treatment is not provided, it may result in blindness.

What to Look for

- Pain, watering eye or redness in the eye.
- Cloudy vision and headaches (glaucoma).
- Sudden loss of vision.
- Limited eye movements.
- Eyelids stuck together (bacterial conjunctivitis).
- Blood on the surface of the eyeball.

What to Do

- For irritation caused by foreign objects or toxic chemicals, immediately and slowly rinse with tap water at room temperature. Rinse from the side to avoid pouring water on the pupil itself, then call 999.
- Call 999 if the patient suffers a sudden loss of vision. Specialized eye centres are better equipped to handle ophthalmic emergencies caused by chemical or physical trauma, infections or dislodged contact lenses.

What Not to Do

- Don't try to remove objects from the eye because you could scratch the cornea.
- Don't pour water directly on the pupil.

Typical Treatment

Minor problems (foreign objects, conjunctivitis and chemical exposure) can be treated in most A&E units, where staff will examine the retina and optic nerve for haemorrhages, retinal detachment and optic neuritis (a possible sign of multiple sclerosis). The front of the cornea is stained with dye so examinations with specialized lenses can detect abrasions.

A patient with a retinal emergency, an acute form of glaucoma or internal haemorrhage due to diabetes should receive immediate, specialized testing, which may not be available at many small hospitals. These patients should be rushed to a designated eye care facility, where accurate diagnosis, administration of eye drops, intravenous medication (mannitol or acetazolamide for glaucoma) or surgery may be needed to prevent permanent vision loss. When a stroke is suspected, a patient's vital signs will be checked and stabilized and ECG, echocardiograms, carotid ultrasound scans, CT scans or an MRI may be performed.

Antibiotic eye drops are prescribed for bacterial infections. Topical antibiotics are also prescribed for corneal abrasions and the eye may be temporarily patched.

After-care

Conjunctivitis and foreign object injuries usually heal within 48 hours and leave no permanent damage. After initial treatment, get a quick check-up from the ophthalmologist (eye specialist) to make sure that no complications arose and that the cornea wasn't scratched. Corneal abrasions can become infected and scar, so a patient should continue taking antibiotics and see an eye specialist regularly for several weeks to monitor the healing. The tiny broken blood vessels that cause subconjunctival haemorrhages usually take about two weeks to heal.

A patient whose vision was compromised by circulatory or cardiac problems will be given echocardiograms and/or Doppler ultrasound scan to check the circulation in the main blood vessels of the neck and heart. If the patient has unstable atrial fibrillation or critically narrowed neck arteries, the blood should be thinned with aspirin, warfarin, heparin or other anticoagulant.

Doctor Says

Vision occurs when patterns of light, colour, shape and movement are projected through the pupil onto the retina. From there, neurochemical impulses are transmitted through the optic nerve, where they ultimately reach the visual processing centre in the brain. In accident and emergency units, the phrase 'curtain up' is bad news because it means retinal detachment.

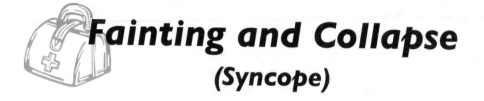

Fainting and Collapse
(Syncope)

What Are They

Fainting occurs when we suddenly and briefly lose consciousness. The oxygen supply to our brain is temporarily impaired; we then lose muscle control of our legs and collapse. Collapse is a protective mechanism because the blood flow to the head is more easily restored when patients are lying down.

Heart problems such as a slowed pulse (which may require a pacemaker), rhythm disturbances (such as atrial fibrillation) and structural abnormalities (defective or rigid valves) that reduce the normal blood flow can cause a sudden collapse. Fainting and collapse can be caused by severe bacterial infections, anaemia, diarrhoea, dehydration and heat exposure. Either can also be the side effect of various antihypertensive and cardiac medications (diuretics, beta-blockers). None of these conditions can be diagnosed or treated at home.

Fainting can be caused by episodes of intense emotion such as fear or stress. During these episodes, the heart will race and then abruptly slow, reducing blood pressure and causing the patient to collapse.

What to Look for

- Paleness.
- Cool and clammy skin.

- Complaints of dizziness or light-headedness.
- Dimmed vision.
- Unsteady gait.
- Falling or collapsing.

What to Do

All patients

- Immediately place the patient flat on his/her back with knees pointing towards the ceiling and soles of the feet flat on the ground. Place a cool, wet cloth on the patient's forehead. See if he/she is conscious (ask 'Are you okay?') and check for a pulse.
- If the patient is unconscious, has no pulse or doesn't respond to your question, first call 999 and then immediately begin CPR (see page 192). Check for a pulse by feeling the inside of the wrist at the point closest to the thumb with fingers other than your thumb. Ideally, the patient will have a steady pulse of about one heart beat per second (see page 190).
- If the patient is conscious, has a strong pulse and says he/she feels better, keep the patient lying down for at least ten minutes, even if they want to rise.

Elderly patients

Call 999 immediately because the patient's collapse may be due to heart disease or the side effects of medication. See if the patient is conscious, check for a pulse and ask if he/she is okay. If the patient is unconscious, has no pulse or doesn't respond to your question, first call 999 and then immediately begin CPR (see page 192). Stay with the patient until emergency personnel arrive.

Young patients

Some patients commonly have episodes called vasovagal syncope, especially during emotional or frightening experiences. These look like serious cardiovascular emergencies, but will last for only a few minutes and then improve. In such instances, place the patient on his/her back with the legs or knees elevated slightly. Check for a pulse in the wrist. To begin with, you'll probably feel a slow pulse (40 to 50 beats per minute) while the patient comes to. If the patient is conscious, has a strong, steady pulse and says that he/she feels better, keep the patient lying flat for at least ten minutes, even if he/she insists on getting up.

What Not to Do

Don't check the pulse or blood pressure until the patient is lying down in the position described above. Otherwise, he/she might collapse while you are checking his/her vital signs and incur additional injuries.

Typical Treatment

A&E staff will usually try to determine the cause of the collapse from the history of the event, a physical examination, lab tests (for anaemia or dehydration) and an ECG (this will detect heart block or other rhythm disturbances). If the collapse was the result of stress or anxiety, treatment is usually unnecessary except for treating injuries caused by the fall.

The patient is usually monitored in A&E for several hours and is not released unless the vital signs have stabilized. Longer observation, or even hospitalization, may be ordered for a patient with heart or circulatory ailments.

After-care

Usually, no further treatment or testing is necessary, unless cardiovascular disease is suspected. If heart problems are responsible for the episode, a consulting cardiologist will decide which tests to order. The options available include an echocardiogram, a stress test and a 24-hour heart monitor.

Doctor Says

Patients who faint often say, 'I want to get better on my own.' However, it is best to treat them as though they are seriously ill rather than minimizing the symptoms. Anxiety is a common cause of fainting. Doctors and nurses frequently encounter patients who start to pass out the moment they see a hypodermic needle coming at them. In fact, some people even get woozy when they see injections in movies.

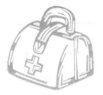

Fractures

What They Are

Simply put, fractures are breaks in bones. Open (compound) fractures are breaks in which bone is exposed through the skin. This creates an opening for contamination and infection. Fractures are also classified by the part of the bone injured (for example, mid-shaft fractures), by the shape of the break (spiral fractures) and how the disrupted segments relate to each other (displaced or nondisplaced fractures). They are often accompanied by sprains (damage to ligaments that connect one bone to another), strains (injuries to tendons, the fibres that attach muscles to bones) or bruises (pockets of blood in connective tissues).

Car accidents can cause fractures to any of the seven vertebrae of the neck (cervical spine). They occur when cars suddenly decelerate and the passenger's neck continues its forward movement. If bone fragments injure nerves in the spinal cord, accident victims may be permanently paralysed.

Patients who extend their arms to break falls often sustain arm and wrist fractures, ligament tears and dislocations. Dislocations occur when the bones in a joint (the pivot point of two adjoining bones) are forced out of the joint, causing immobility and pain.

The elderly are prone to fractures of the hip joint because of their unsteadiness and fragile bones. Children incur two unique types of injuries: greenstick fractures (incomplete breaks that rarely need surgery) and damage to the growth plate at the ends of developing long bones.

What to Look for

- Abnormally shaped arm or leg bones.
- Protruding bones.
- Extreme pain.
- Bruises.
- Swelling.
- Brown urine, a sign of massive muscle injury.

What to Do

- Call 999 immediately. Emergency medical personnel will stabilize the injured area and then transport the patient for additional care. They will also check for damage to patient's nerves, arteries or veins and, in the case of rib fractures, lungs and heart, which may require more immediate attention than the fractures themselves.
- Check that the patient has an open airway, stable breathing and a pulse, even when their injuries don't seem to involve critical organs. Unseen internal chest and abdominal trauma (bleeding around the lungs, ruptured spleen) may accompany serious orthopaedic injuries.
- Cover exposed bone fragments with clean gauze to minimize exposure to bacterial contamination.
- Elevate and apply cold compresses to the injured area.

What Not to Do

- Don't move or touch a patient with neck injuries! Wait for the ambulance! The smallest movements can cause spinal cord damage. Emergency personnel will transport neck injury patients on specialized boards or in a brace that will immobilize their necks.

- Don't let a patient with a hip injury walk. Although a patient with a nondisplaced hip fracture may be able to bear weight, doing so could then cause displacement and further injury.
- Don't move fractured bones or allow others to move them. The sharp edges of fractured bones could pierce adjacent tissue, injuring nerves and blood vessels and/or piercing the skin. Instead, move both ends of the fractured bone simultaneously as a unit and place them in a straight line. If possible, immobilize the fracture (see page 203). Emergency medical personnel should perform this task unless, of course, no ambulance service is available.

Typical Treatment

Emergency personnel will first check and stabilize the patient's vital signs. Then they will try to make the patient more comfortable and, when possible, place the fractured bone segments in alignment (reducing the fracture). They will try to align the bone as close to its original position as possible because bone tissue is continuously active and will 'recognize' and unite with a separated piece. Alignment facilitates healing and in healing, the bone will hopefully replicate its original structure.

In A&E, X-rays will be taken to ascertain the extent of injury and determine whether surgery is needed. All orthopaedic injuries will be compared to the unaffected side of the body. However, children frequently have both affected and unaffected limbs X-rayed so that a normal, growing bone is not mistaken for a fracture.

Broken limbs are often immobilized with plaster or fibreglass casts (closed reduction). Special supports may be used used for fractures of the shoulder, collar bone, arm, hand, knee and ankle.

Bleeding deep inside the hand, arm or leg may inhibit normal circulation. When tissues cannot stretch to accommodate the increased fluid, muscles and nerves may be compressed (a compartment syndrome). Patients will feel numbness of the skin directly over the injured area and the injured limb will be pale, painful and/or immobile. Immediate surgery is often required to relieve the compression and save the affected tissues.

Shoulder dislocations are usually corrected by manually moving displaced bone back into the joint. But other dislocations, such as those to a hip, may require surgical repair. Breaks of the collar bone, nose, ribs, pelvis and shoulder blades are usually allowed to heal on their own. Simple, nondisplaced fractures that are stabilized in casts are X-rayed over the following few weeks to monitor healing. Strains, sprains and bruises that accompany fractures are also treated in A&E, usually with cold compresses and elevation to minimize tissue swelling.

Severe injury to an arm, leg, or hip may require surgery (open reduction) within 24 hours. If the injury involves an open fracture, immediate surgery (and intravenous antibiotics) will be needed. Cervical spine fractures, especially when unstable, require prompt evaluation with CT scanning, MRI and neurosurgery.

A healed fracture site may become stronger than the original bone because the healing process often lays down extra new bone.

Common orthopaedic emergencies include:

1. Fracture of the fifth metacarpal bone of the hand ('boxer's fracture').
2. Collar bone fracture (the most common fracture of childhood).
3. Colles' fracture (of the forearm at the wrist).
4. Pelvic fracture (often resulting in internal haemorrhage).
5. Anterior dislocation of the shoulder (treated with manipulation).
6. Rotator cuff injury (inflammation or rupture of shoulder muscles, restricting arm raising or overhead movements).
7. Hip fracture (producing shortening and outward rotation of the leg).

8. Sprain of outer ankle ligaments (the most common ankle injury).
9. Dislocation of elbow (also due to falls, it may injure nerves and blood vessels if not quickly identified and treated).

After-care

Most orthopaedic injuries do not require hospitalization, but an orthopaedic surgeon (bone specialist) should see the patient every few days until the swelling and pain begin to disappear. Orthopaedic surgeons periodically re-examine and may X-ray and recast patients. Patients who have not had surgery generally make a good recovery.

Patients who cannot walk without assistance will need a wheelchair, cane or crutches. At home, the injured limb must initially be elevated above heart level. For example, if a patient's leg is broken, he/she should lie down with the leg raised so accumulated tissue fluid and blood can flow 'downhill'.

After surgery, patients with major vertebral or spinal fractures will remain in the hospital several days or even weeks. When their conditions stabilize, they will be transferred to a rehabilitation facility, where they will remain for several more weeks to recuperate. Seriously infected open fractures (osteomyelitis) require intravenous antibiotics, often for a month or more.

Doctor Says

Even when X-rays are taken immediately after an injury, several types of fracture can be missed. A patient who experiences pain and discomfort within seven to ten days needs a follow-up orthopaedic examination. Fractures frequently missed include those to the elbow (radial head), foot ('stress' or 'march') and wrist (navicular).

Again, don't move anyone who has neck pain after an accident, especially a high-impact injury. Don't even touch them. Wait for qualified emergency medical personnel!

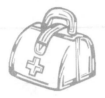

Gunshot and Stab Wounds

What They Are

Direct, blunt trauma and shock waves from high-velocity bullets will damage everything in their path. Bullets enter the body in a spinning, twisting motion and will break bones, rupture internal organs and shred muscles. Tissues adjoining a wound may stretch, detach or be torn from heat, metal or bone fragments. A victim's outward appearance may be deceiving because internal injuries may not be apparent to untrained observers.

On the other hand, the damage from a low-velocity knife or a small-calibre bullet wound is usually more apparent and localized. Victims usually incur noticeable wounds and bleeding. Perforation of a single critical organ, such as the spleen or a lung, may have rapid, fatal consequences. A severed and exposed artery anywhere in the body can create potentially deadly blood loss.

Distressingly, it is the case that penetrating wounds caused by knives, bullets and broken bottles are a growing problem in the UK, accounting for an increasing number of A&E visits.

What to Look for

- A penetrating wound.
- Localized pain.
- Bleeding.
- Pale, cold and clammy skin (from blood loss, which may be internal).

- Dizziness, unsteadiness or collapse.
- Shortness of breath, particularly when a chest injury causes a lung to deflate.

Gunshot victims, especially those in their twenties or thirties, may not show any outward signs of severe internal bleeding. Whenever you find a penetrating wound to the chest below the nipples, assume that the patient has an abdominal injury.

What to Do
- Call 999 immediately. Speed is of the essence.
- Keep the victim lying down, calm and quiet. Otherwise, a patient who is bleeding internally could faint and incur further injuries.

First Aid
1. Pack the wound with clean gauze pads.

2. Apply direct pressure with a clean cloth, dressing or gauze on a bleeding wound to stop the blood flow. But do not delay while looking for a clean dressing – the priority is to stop the flow of blood.

3. If direct pressure to an arm or leg wound fails to stop the bleeding, feel for the pulse on the inner side of the upper arm (brachial artery) or top of the leg near the groin (femoral artery) and apply pressure there.

What Not to Do
- Don't try to remove a bullet or knife. A lodged weapon may be preventing blood loss. Removal could expose a severed artery or vein, leading to circulatory collapse.
- Don't scrub the area or use soaps of any kind.

- Don't allow the patient to stand, walk or eat.
- Don't elevate a bleeding arm or leg because an artery may be injured and circulation of blood to the limb could be impaired.
- Don't make any assumptions about the extent of the patient's injury because a bullet's path is unpredictable. Get the patient immediate treatment.

Typical Treatment

Stabilizing the patient's vital signs is always the first priority. While doing so, the A&E staff will assess the extent of the injuries. Treatment can range from cleaning and stitching the patient's wound to complex surgery, depending on the extent of the injury.

Seriously injured patients may be taken to specialized trauma centres, where surgical teams are on hand. The precise treatment they provide will depend on the organs affected, the extent of the damage and the pathway that the weapon created.

Since skin bacteria (staphylococci, for example) are pushed into the deeper connective tissues during a bullet or knife injury, patients are usually treated with antibiotics for at least one week.

After-care

Hospital staff will provide specific instructions consistent with the injuries. The wounds should be re-examined within four to seven days after the original treatment or hospital discharge, at which time most stitches can be removed. Antibiotics are usually continued for about two weeks.

Doctor Says

Consider all gunshot and stab wounds to be potentially fatal. An apparently minor abdominal wound might result in a ruptured spleen, leading to internal haemorrhage and shock. Young patients (the most likely victims) may lose as much as 60 per cent of their blood internally without showing outward signs of injury.

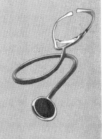

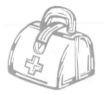

Headaches

What They Are

Although virtually everyone gets headaches, most of them are minor and over-the-counter pain remedies usually provide quick relief. However, some headaches are long-lasting, resistant to pain remedies and indicate serious medical problems that require prompt treatment.

No one knows what causes some of the most common types of headache, but a number of theories exist. Headaches can be attributable to the misfiring or overstimulation of pain receptors in the skull or a heightened sensitivity to normal arterial pulsations. They may also be due to high blood pressure, sinusitis, dental disease, eye (glaucoma), ear and neck ailments and alcohol intoxication (hangovers) to name but a few. Headaches can cause intense pain, but they usually don't produce any visible physical abnormalities. Only about 4 per cent of all headaches result from damage to internal structures in the skull.

What to Look for

Cluster headaches

- Short bouts of pain around one eye (can waken patient from sleep).
- Intense anxiety and agitation.
- Redness around the eye (a 'shiner'), watering eyes and a runny nose.

Headaches

Migraine headaches
- An 'aura' of flashing lights, dark spots or jagged lines may precede the attack.
- Throbbing pain on one side of the skull that may last for hours or, in extreme cases, days.
- Sensitivity to bright lights or loud sounds.

Tension headaches
- Constricting pain, 'like a knot' or like muscle spasms, over the patient's entire scalp or neck.
- Pain worsening with stress as the day progresses.

Traction headaches
- Sudden onset.
- Disorientation, unresponsiveness or unconsciousness.
- Nausea and vomiting.
- Pain caused by abnormal collections of blood that compress brain tissue. These include intracranial bleeding (cerebral aneurysms, subdural haematoma and subarachnoid haemorrhage), haemorrhagic strokes and expanding mass lesions such as brain tumours.

Temporal Arteritis
- Pain on one side of forehead.
- Impaired vision or blindness affecting the eye on the same side as the pain.

Infections of the brain (encephalitis) or its covering membranes (meningitis)

- Fever.
- Nausea, vomiting.
- Stiffness of the neck.
- Confusion and delirium.

What to Do

- Call 999 immediately if the patient has neck stiffness, vomits or becomes unresponsive – time is of the essence.
- Call 999 immediately if the patient is dizzy, unsteady, confused or having the 'worst headache I've ever felt'. Violent headaches that begin suddenly may indicate bleeding into the brain.
- Treat mild headaches that are not accompanied by other symptoms with over-the-counter painkillers (paracetamol and codeine) or anti-inflammatory drugs (aspirin or ibuprofen), bed rest in a quiet, dark environment and cold compresses to the forehead.
- Notify the patient's doctor of newly developing headaches or changes in the usual pattern.

Typical Treatment

Often, the patient's symptoms may not accurately identify the actual headache syndrome involved. For example, a migraine can appear to be a tension headache or encephalitis may resemble a cluster headache. Therefore, the A&E staff will base treatment more on patient history than on the 'textbook' signs.

Patients will be questioned about the onset, location, severity, duration and frequency of their pain, and also any associated symptoms (nausea, vomiting, dizziness, auras, double vision, fever or neck stiffness) and the precipitating factors (medications, foods, exertion or wine).

The most serious headaches, those associated with brain tumours or with bleeding into the central nervous system, are identified by diagnostic CT scans or MRI. These serious conditions usually require complex neurosurgery to prevent respiratory arrest and death. On rare occasions, small holes are drilled into the skull to relieve pressure.

When meningitis is suspected, a lumbar puncture will be performed. The patient's spinal fluid will be examined. Antibiotic or antiviral medications will usually be started before test results come back.

Cluster headaches, unlike other headaches, often improve when patients receive extremely high concentrations of oxygen.

When the cause of the headache is diagnosed, a variety of medications can be prescribed to address the specific type of headache. These include beta-blockers, anti-inflammatory drugs and over-the-counter remedies. Fluid replacement and rest in a quiet, dark room are also helpful.

Patients with temporal arteritis will be given corticosteroids.

After-care

Migraine, cluster headaches and temporal arteritis are chronic conditions that feature relapses and pain-free intervals. In addition to over-the-counter remedies, a variety of medications are prescribed for specific headache syndromes. These include ergotamine, lithium, beta-blockers and anti-inflammatory drugs. Usually, a patient begins taking these drugs in the A&E unit. Several days later, during an examination by the patient's GP, the effectiveness of the medication and its dosage will be evaluated.

If the patient is required to take medication regularly to remain pain-free, his/her doctor should be seen at least every four to six weeks to monitor the condition and medication.

Doctor Says

High blood pressure does not usually cause headaches. However, headaches may cause raised blood pressure. Severe headaches in a burn victim can indicate carbon monoxide poisoning.

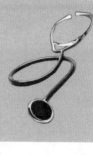

Head Injuries

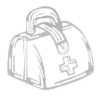

What They Are

Trauma to the skull can damage or destroy brain cells and cause intracranial bleeding. Severe trauma can also cause fractures of the skull itself. Head injuries can occur during car crashes or violent attacks, but they can also follow seemingly minor injuries.

Internal swelling from head injuries can cause compression of the brain stem, the control centre that regulates most of our important bodily functions. Brain stem compression can damage the respiratory centre and cause death by paralysing the diaphragm (the muscle between the abdomen and chest that enables us to breathe).

Blunt skull trauma results from blows to the head, such as those incurred during sporting events or falls. Such trauma can cause concussion, the brief loss of consciousness that may be accompanied by memory loss. Injuries associated with concussions can cause permanent brain damage, so patients who lose consciousness should receive prompt medical care.

WARNING: Seemingly mild head injuries can turn into serious problems within 24 hours (in rare cases, even as long as a month later). Patients over 65, especially those taking blood-thinning medication, run greater risks of complications.

What to Look for

- Brief loss of consciousness.
- Inability to remember what occurred.
- Headache.

- Dizziness.
- Confusion.
- Arm or leg weakness or unsteadiness.
- Speech impairment.
- Sleepiness.

What to Do

- Ask the patient's name, what day it is and where he/she is.
- If the response is not correct, call 999 immediately.
- Patients with chronic medical conditions, especially those with hypertension and heart ailments, should be taken for prompt emergency evaluation.
- Look for blood or clear fluid in the nose or ears (often a sign of a skull fracture).
- Unequal pupil size may indicate brain stem compression.

What Not to Do

Don't give sedatives. They could complicate diagnosis and cause dangerous respiratory problems.

Typical Treatment

A&E medical personnel will document and monitor the patient's vital signs, orientation, bodily movements, ability to follow instructions and speech pattern.

When the brain's respiratory centre is injured, proper blood flow will be restored using mechanical respiration. The patient's blood pressure and pulse will be checked to determine if internal injuries such as spleen rupture or intra-abdominal bleeding were suffered. If so, intravenous fluids, medication or surgery may be necessary.

If CT scans detect intracranial bleeding, holes will be drilled into the skull to drain haematomas (areas of swelling due to collected blood). Draining is intended to alleviate intracranial pressure and avoid damage to the respiratory centre. Cerebral compression frequently triggers a reflex that slows the pulse. If that occurs, patients will be fitted with a cardiac pacemaker.

Surgery is performed on fractured skulls only if the brain has been compressed by bone fragments (a 'depressed' skull fracture).

After-care

Older patients, especially those who live alone, will usually be hospitalized and monitored for at least 24 hours. Young, healthy patients without concussion or amnesia are usually sent home after initial treatment, but their family and friends should monitor their conditions for at least the next 24 hours. If they show any of the symptoms described above, they should immediately return to the hospital.

Doctor Says

Usually, impaired thinking, concentration and memory caused by head injuries improve within a few months. Some patients may continue to have minor headaches, insomnia and depression even though their tests reveal no abnormalities. If so, avoid medications that might disguise potentially important symptoms.

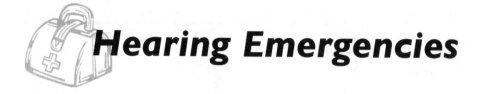# *Hearing Emergencies*

What They Are

Our ears are built to capture sound waves and funnel them to our eardrums. The captured sound waves are turned into vibrations that flow through the auditory canal to small internal bones and receptors that convert the vibrations into impulses that the brain decodes. Interruption of this process at any point can distort, muffle or even eliminate those sounds.

The eardrum is susceptible to injury from accidents (from diving, foreign objects and direct blows), infection and from incorrect cleaning (inserting cotton wool swabs too deeply). Swimmer's ear (otitis externa) is similar to a skin infection and is usually caused by common skin bacteria (staphylococcus and pseudomonas). Infection in the central auditory canal (otitis media) occurs when upper respiratory tract infections spread through the mouth and eustachian tube into one ear.

The inner ear controls not only our hearing, but also our balance. Nerve connections between the inner ear and the eye muscles (via the brain) enable us to coordinate vision and balance. An infection of the inner ear is called acute labyrinthitis and is usually a complication of a cold. It produces severe vertigo (misperception of movement when an individual is motionless) and imbalance, not hearing loss.

Ménière's disease is characterized by repeated episodes of vertigo, hearing loss, ringing in the ears and a 'stuffed-up' feeling. It can be a recurrent condition that lasts for decades.

The most common cause of impaired hearing occurs when thick gobs of earwax accumulate and plug the eardrum. The wax blocks the passage of sound waves to the eardrum – just like a muted trumpet. Wax can be removed easily at your GP's surgery and treatment at an acute-care facility is not necessary.

What to Look for

- *Eardrum perforations (punctures).* Intense pain in the ear, bloody drainage, dizziness, ringing sounds and/or hearing loss.
- *Trapped objects* in the ear, such as beans, cotton wool swab tips, insects and even earwax. Often, when patients try to remove objects, they push them in more deeply. To prevent infection, irritation or perforation, have only trained medical personnel remove foreign objects.
- *Swimmer's ear* (otitis externa). Yellow secretions draining from the ear, pain when opening the mouth widely and often fever.
- *Middle ear infection* (otitis media). Children tugging an ear, adults experiencing hearing loss, earache, fever and watery discharge. In severe middle ear infections, eardrums bulge outwardly (from a build-up of inflammatory secretions) and can then go on to perforate.
- *Inner ear infection* (labyrinthitis). Complaints that 'the room is spinning', nausea and vomiting, but no hearing loss.

What to Do

- See your GP immediately or go to a walk-in centre or hospital accident and emergency unit.
- If children tug at one ear or adults have hearing loss, earache, fever and watery discharge (middle ear infection), see your GP at once.

What Not to Do

- Don't remove foreign objects. You may infect, irritate, or perforate the eardrum. Have a healthcare professional do it!
- You do not normally need to call 999 for ear disorders.

Typical Treatment

When an eardrum is perforated but the tiny receptors in the middle ear are not damaged, further treatment usually isn't needed. The doctor will rinse out the ear, prescribe antibiotic drops and may schedule a follow-up examination in a few days. Up to 90 per cent of perforations heal by themselves in three to four months, but serious perforations require hospitalization, intravenous antibiotics and surgery.

Removing foreign objects from children's ears often requires sedation. Trapped insects can be drowned by gently washing the ear with lidocaine solution or olive oil.

Swimmer's ear is usually eliminated when topical antibiotics are applied with a medicine dropper several times a day. Normally, no follow-up is necessary.

Middle ear infections are treated with oral antibiotics (amoxicillin or erythromycin), the same drugs prescribed for bronchitis and lung infections.

Labyrinthitis responds well to meclozine. However, since vertigo may recur (especially in Ménière's disease), it is important for a patient to quickly spot the symptoms and take meclozine to minimize the attacks.

After-care

For perforated eardrums, patients should take antibiotic drops and be re-examined several days later to monitor healing.

Middle ear infections should be checked a week after initial treatment to make sure that the structures in the auditory canal and hearing were not affected.

Doctor Says

Working at the Emergency Room (ER) at New York City's Cabrini Hospital, I once treated a child who was plagued by a 'buzzing in one ear'. Imagine my shock when I looked through the otoscope and saw a cockroach staring straight back at me. The intruder was quickly dislodged with a mineral oil bath.

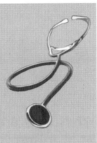

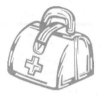

Heart Attacks

What They Are

When an artery carrying blood to the heart is blocked, the heart muscle is suddenly deprived of vital oxygen. Without oxygen, heart-muscle cells can die. When they die, the heart cannot pump blood throughout the body effectively, depriving crucial organs such as the brain and kidneys of the oxygen and nutrients they need to survive. Microscopic electrical misfirings can be triggered in the heart (arrhythmias). Blood and tissue fluid can accumulate in the lungs and legs (congestive heart failure).

The term 'acute coronary syndrome' refers to diseases ranging from mild, chronic chest pains (angina pectoris) to deadly heart attacks (myocardial infarctions). Heart attacks claim around 150,000 deaths in the UK annually.

What to Look for

- Left-sided chest pain, central chest pain ('like an elephant standing on me'), central abdominal pain, jaw or neck pain or left shoulder pain that may travel down the back of either or both arms.
- Heart attack pain lasts up to two hours. Pain due to chronic angina, which is provoked by exertion and relieved by rest, lasts 2–20 minutes. Exercise, cold weather and stress can also cause chest pain.
- Possible nausea, vomiting, shortness of breath, palpitations, severe dizziness or cold sweat on the forehead.

WARNING: *Heart attacks can occur without any of the above symptoms, especially in women.*

What to Do

- Call 999 immediately. Speed is of the essence. Quick action saves most heart attack victims.
- Take the patient's pulse to determine its strength (see page 190). If the patient has ho pulse, perform CPR (see page 192).
- If the patient has glyceryl trinitrate (for angina), insert or spray it under the tongue.
- Give the patient a single aspirin (of at least 160mg).

What Not to Do

Don't delay calling 999 for even a second, even if the patient has sudden cardiac arrest!

Typical Treatment

Monitored hospital confinement is needed for at least two to three days. Two tests confirm the diagnosis: the electrocardiogram, which shows the electrical damage done to heart muscle, and blood tests, which identify chemicals released from dead heart cells.

Medications that will be given include intravenous glyceryl trinitrate to open unaffected blood vessels, morphine for severe pain, beta-blockers to relax and slow the heart and nasal oxygen to keep jeopardized cells alive.

During a heart attack, the patient's blood stream becomes thicker and stickier. Therefore, intravenous fluids and medications (heparin, streptokinase, alteplase) are administered to thin blood and/or destroy large blood clots.

Strict bed rest is needed until the crisis passes.

Critically ill patients may need coronary blockages opened by high-tech surgery in which clogged arteries are burrowed through (angioplasty) or replaced by a blood vessel (coronary bypass surgery) usually taken from the patient's leg or chest wall. A stainless-steel tube (stent) is inserted to open the affected artery, to keep it open and to restore normal circulation.

After-care

Cardiac patients must begin a lifetime regimen to address their bad habits (obesity, smoking, lack of physical exercise) and tackle these adverse risk factors (through changes in diet, giving up smoking, taking exercise and starting stress management).

Patients will be put on medication, including glyceryl trinitrate and cholesterol-lowering drugs (statins) and/or blood pressure drugs (antihypertensives).

Most nonsurgical patients stabilize and improve within three weeks. Recovery period for surgery patients depends on the extent and nature of the surgery.

Doctor Says

Two-thirds of heart-attack patients survive with prompt treatment. It's better to err on the side of caution and assume that any severe chest symptom represents a cardiac emergency. Learn how to take a pulse and practise on family and friends. Learn CPR as well!

Heart Rhythm Abnormalities

What They Are

Our organs, tissues and cells need oxygen to survive. They get oxygen from blood that circulates through the body; the supply must be regular and uninterrupted. Normally, an adult heart pumps blood in a steady, even pattern between 50 to 100 beats per minute (bpm). When the heart rate is less than 40bpm or over 150bpm, the supply of blood that the heart circulates can decrease. Either abnormality can lower blood pressure significantly because the heart doesn't fill up properly.

Some patients experience 'extra heartbeats', sporadic twitching of irritable heart-muscle fibres. Although these are common and usually harmless, extra heartbeats can impair circulation leading to dizziness and collapse.

When unusually large electrical disturbances spread through cardiac muscle, the heart literally stops pumping and brain cells will begin to die within three to five minutes. These disturbances can come on suddenly without warning or clue.

Abnormal or disordered electrical flow can cause ineffective pumping in the atria (the two upper heart chambers) or the ventricles (the two lower heart chambers). Ventricular fibrillation (muscle fibre twitching and wiggling) will usually paralyse the heart muscle and must be treated immediately.

In addition, both the upper and lower heart chambers can become electrically independent of each other, which is called heart block. More common, but less deadly, are extremely rapid impulses generated during upper-heart (atrial) fibrillation, during which the heart rate may be over 200bpm.

What to Look for

- Irregular, chaotic, or extremely rapid heartbeats (palpitations).
- Shortness of breath.
- Chest pain.
- Dizziness, light-headedness.
- Dimmed vision.
- Collapse.

What to Do

- Call 999 immediately and say, 'This is a cardiac emergency.'
- Check the patient's pulse to determine the heart rate (see page 190). Heart rates can be influenced by the patient's age, temperature, emotions, level of fitness and hormonal chemistry. For example, an athlete's resting pulse may be 30–40bpm, while an infant's is usually 130–160. Pay more attention to the symptoms listed above than to the patient's pulse rate.
- Give CPR (see page 192) when the patient isn't breathing and the heart isn't beating. If ventricular (lower heart) tachycardia is suspected, thump the patient once sharply on the breastbone as if you were pounding on a door.

Typical Treatment

When a patient's heart has stopped, emergency medical personnel will try to revive him/her by giving CPR and/or applying electrical current directly to the chest wall. In less critical situations, emergency personnel will try to stabilize the patient to make sure that blood flows continuously to the brain and heart. A patient being transported to the hospital will be given oxygen and possibly intravenous medication (lidocaine or atropine) to either slow, speed up, or normalize the heartbeat pattern.

At the accident and emergency unit, the patient will be given an ECG and receive continuous cardiac monitoring. The precise treatment will depend primarily on the patient's circulatory condition as well as the nature and rate of the rhythm disturbance itself.

A patient who has a very slow heart rate (usually under 50bpm) will receive a pacemaker – an implanted, battery-driven, electronic device that stimulates the heart so that it beats effectively.

To control heart rhythm disturbances, intravenous medications (digitalis, beta-blockers, quinidine, calcium-channel antagonists and lidocaine) may be administered. These medications are injected slowly over several hours while the patient's response and vital signs are monitored.

Most patients with heart-rhythm disturbances will be kept under close observation for at least 24 hours. Those with more serious or unstable conditions will remain in the intensive care unit for at least a few days.

After-care

Periodic evaluation by a cardiologist is a must! Some patients will be required to continue taking stabilizing medication (propranolol, verapamil, digitalis, quinidine) for the rest of their lives. Patients with underlying coronary disease should be given stress tests, echocardiograms or home monitoring to prevent recurrences that could prove more dangerous than the initial attack.

Doctor Says

Up to 25 per cent of all deaths from heart disorders – over 150,000 annually – are caused by electrical-flow disturbances. In evaluating a patient, assessing whether blood is circulating properly is more important than the patient's heart rhythm. Blood pressure collapse, which results from cardiac arrest and shock, can be caused by fast, slow or chaotic heartbeat. Call 999 if this is suspected.

Heat Emergencies
(Hyperthermia)

What They Are

Our cells die at temperatures of around 45°C (113°F) and never regenerate. Therefore, we have developed mechanisms that operate like thermostats to regulate our body temperature. When we get too hot, warm body fluids are sent to pores on the skin's surface, where they evaporate as sweat. Conversely, we shiver when we are cold to generate muscle heat in the blood that warms our tissues.

Problems arise when the body can't rid itself of excess heat. During periods of high humidity, the body retains heat because sweat does not fully evaporate. In addition, the body cannot eliminate all excessive heat caused by infection (fever), hyperactivity (epilepsy, alcohol withdrawal), certain drug use (cocaine, PCP and amphetamines) and prolonged exposure (saunas, hot baths and overheated cars).

Sports enthusiasts or outdoor workers can lose too much fluid sweating in hot, humid weather and become dehydrated. Dehydration – the loss of too much body fluid and salt – decreases blood pressure and causes symptoms ranging from mild, uncomfortable heat cramps to painful muscle spasms (in the arms, legs or upper torso), severe headache and two potentially dangerous conditions: heatstroke and heat exhaustion.

Heatstroke occurs when the brain's thermostat is disrupted and body temperature rises above 40°C (104.9°F). Instead of losing heat and cooling off, heatstroke patients become hotter, paradoxically, often to levels that are warmer than their surroundings. When body temperature is not regulated, a patient's vital organ functions can be severely damaged. Frail, elderly patients, infants and the economically deprived are especially prone to heatstroke.

Heat exhaustion is essentially severe dehydration that seldom requires hospitalization. Although it can cause damage to the heart, brain or kidneys, patients usually recover fully.

What to Look for

- Altered mental state. Disorientation or delirium (sign of heatstroke).
- Flushed, reddened skin.
- Dry, hot skin that may be warmer than the outside temperature (sign of heatstroke).
- Total unresponsiveness (heatstroke).
- Leg muscle cramps.
- Severe headache.

What to Do

- Before calling 999, move the patient out of direct sunlight to a cool, shady spot, if possible.
- Call 999 if the patient has heatstroke. Suspect heatstroke when the patient's skin is warmer than the outside temperature – often over 40.5°C (105°F) – or if the patient is delirious, disoriented or unresponsive (comatose).
- Remove or open constricting clothing.
- Sponge cold water liberally on the skin and fan the patient.
- Gently massage the limbs to promote circulation and prevent tissue damage in the fingers and toes.
- Give water to patients with leg cramps, but do make sure that they drink it slowly. When emergency medical personnel arrive, they will be able to administer intravenous fluids.

What Not to Do

- Don't try to cool heatstroke patients by giving them cold beverages or food; their digestion may be impaired and they could vomit or choke.
- Don't allow an overheated patient to stand or walk on his/her own. The lower blood volume caused by dehydration may cause him/her to collapse.
- Don't give patients salt tablets, because they need immediate fluid replacement.
- Don't give patients aspirin or ibuprofen, which are not helpful for heat-related emergencies.

Typical Treatment

Heatstroke is a major medical emergency that can damage many organs. For example, fluid loss and lowered blood pressure may affect tissue oxygenation and cause epileptic seizures, heart rhythm disturbances or kidney problems. Heatstroke can impair the clotting system, damage dehydrated muscle cells and even cause cardiopulmonary arrest.

Since heatstroke can affect many different organs, treatment will vary in accordance with each specific injury. Generally, patients will be cooled with intravenous solutions, ice packs to their armpits and groin and possibly ice water delivered to the stomach via specialized tubing. Unless complications arise, most heatstroke patients will be kept in the intensive care unit for only a few days.

Heat exhaustion patients are usually treated with intravenous fluids and then discharged. However, cardiac patients and the elderly should be monitored for 24 hours after the incident, even if they are feeling better.

After-care

Heat cramps and heat exhaustion usually improve within 24 to 48 hours and rarely require further treatment. When heatstroke is treated promptly, it generally takes at least a week to see significant improvement.

Doctor Says

Assume that a delirious, hot, bone-dry patient has heatstroke until proven otherwise. Heatstroke carries a potentially high risk of mortality because of the catastrophic effects of dehydration and its impact on vital organs.

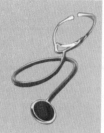

High Blood Pressure

What It Is

When blood circulates through our bodies, it exerts pressure on the inside of our artery walls. In most cases, our bodies operate most efficiently when that pressure ranges between 90/60 and 120/80 (normal readings).

Sustained blood pressure of 180/110 or above can cause strokes, sudden injuries to the brain that may result in paralysis and death. High blood pressure (hypertension) can damage coronary arteries, rupture the aortic wall and cause kidney failure, heart attacks and pulmonary oedema (fluid in the lungs).

Hypertensive encephalopathy, a condition that entails altered levels of consciousness and impaired vision, may occur when blood pressure readings soar to 240/140. Isolated readings that are approximately 10–20 points above normal and that accompany severe pain, panic attacks, stimulant abuse and blood pressure monitoring by doctors ('white coat syndrome') are called transient hypertension.

Although medical science has not been able to identify a definitive cause of high blood pressure, experts believe that the condition may be influenced by dietary indiscretion such as eating too much salt or drinking too much alcohol.

Hypertension can be a silent killer that strikes the unaware. Over half of all those with high blood pressure don't know that they suffer from the disorder.

What to Look for

- Headache, double vision or dizziness.
- Paralysis preventing patients from moving, talking or even breathing (signalling a stroke, the most feared complication).
- Chest pains and palpitations.
- Nausea, vomiting.
- Confusion, disorientation, agitation or sleeplessness.

What to Do

- Call 999 immediately if the patient has double vision, a severe frontal headache, shortness of breath or chest pressure.
- Call 999 when elderly or diabetic people exhibit these symptoms, even if their blood pressure seems normal. Delay can be disastrous.
- A patient suspected of having suffered a heart attack or stroke requires urgent attention regardless of the blood pressure readings.

What Not to Do

Don't give the patient any medication until you clear it with his/her doctor.

Typical Treatment

Emergency treatment focuses on preventing or minimizing damage to the heart, brain and kidneys. Intravenous antihypertensive medications may be administered, such as nitroprusside, labetalol, esmolol or glyceryl trinitrate. For less urgent conditions, oral medications may be given including nifedipine, clonidine and glyceryl trinitrate. Treatment is usually a slow and closely monitored process because lowering blood pressure too quickly can decrease the blood flow to the heart or brain and cause permanent damage.

When hypertensive encephalopathy is promptly treated with intravenous nitroprusside, brain damage can be avoided.

A patient with a high blood pressure emergency is often admitted to a hospital 'for observation'. The person remains hospitalized until his/her blood pressure stabilizes at a safe level (under 140/90) and until tests verify that no cardiovascular, brain or kidney damage has occurred.

After-care

The patient is generally given daily medication. Blood pressure must be monitored at least twice a day and patients – and their carers – should learn how to take blood pressure readings.

Doctor Says

Hypertension is a huge and growing problem that affects 35 per cent of the UK population and over half of senior citizens. Unfortunately, the condition of only about 28 per cent of these people is treated effectively. Have your blood pressure checked regularly and, if it is high, get a home monitor and learn to take accurate readings.

Kidney Stones

What They Are

Kidney stones are pebble-sized pieces of calcium that crystallize in the small tubes of the urinary tract. They often have jagged surfaces or sharp burrs. When these stones can't flow freely 'downstream' from the kidney via the ureter (the tube that conveys urine to the bladder), blockage occurs and causes excruciating pain called renal colic. Kidney stone attacks can be the most painful of all medical emergencies.

Up to 12 per cent of the public will suffer at least one kidney stone attack at some point in their lives. Fortunately, many stones are tiny and smooth so they pass freely and are excreted without complications.

Kidney stone sufferers often lead sedentary lives or reside in dry (desert and mountain) and warm climates.

What to Look for

- A dull ache directly below the ribcage in the left or right mid-back, but not simultaneously on both sides.
- Left or right-sided backache, spreading forward to the lower abdomen and groin.
- Dark, 'rusty-coloured' or brownish urine. Blood in the urine is rare.
- Waves of sudden pain that stop for several minutes, then restart.
- Inability to find a comfortable position (in contrast to peritonitis where patients cannot move).
- Agitation. The patient can't get comfortable in any position so they move around and writhe in pain.

- Nausea, vomiting and sweating.
- Fever and chills if the blockage creates a urinary tract or kidney infection (see Urinary Tract Disorders on page 174).

What to Do

- Call 999.
- Have the patient drink as much water as possible, which may help them pass the stone. However, nausea and vomiting often make drinking fluids impossible.

What Not to Do

Do not give a patient painkillers until hospital testing is completed. Painkillers could disguise crucial symptoms and make diagnosis more difficult.

Typical Treatment

Hospital treatment centres on relieving pain and urinary tract blockage. Medications, including morphine, are injected for pain and intravenous fluids are given to flush out an obstructing stone.

Lower abdominal X-rays (KUB, for kidney-ureter-bladder) may reveal a white 'pebble'. A urinalysis may contain microscopic traces of blood.

Blood tests, including those to detect elevated white blood cell count, can disclose infections that require intravenous antibiotics and hospitalization. If X-rays do not reveal stones, additional tests may be ordered such as ultrasound scans, CT scans or an intravenous urogram (IVU), an hour-long set of X-rays that reveals urinary tract blockage due to a stone that is 'invisible'. A patient will not be discharged until the stone has passed and the patient is infection-free.

During hospitalization, all of the patient's urine is collected over a 24-hour period. This sample will be strained and the sediment retrieved to help identify the stone's constituents. There may be a high concentration of uric acid or abnormal excretion of calcium, citrate and oxalate, any of which can cause kidney stones.

If a kidney stone does not pass within two to three days, the patient's kidneys will be bombarded with sound waves to pulverize the stone into tiny particles that can pass. If sonic bombardment fails, the stone can be surgically removed.

After-care

A patient should see a urologist within several days of hospital discharge, especially if the blockage caused an infection. The patient must continue to dilute his/her urine by drinking at least 3 litres (5 pints) of water each day. The patient may also be required to change his/her diet depending on the findings of the urine analyses. Possible changes include restricting salt, limiting protein, avoiding certain foods (for example, rhubarb, cheese or beer) and taking or avoiding calcium supplements.

Even after a change in diet and increase in fluid intake, kidney stone patients remain at risk of future attacks. Periodic 24-hour urine collections and radiological studies may be required to monitor whether new stones have formed. Patients can also check their urine at home for microscopic traces of blood by using test strips available at most pharmacies.

Doctor Says

Up to 40,00 people are diagnosed with kidney stones each year in the UK. In most cases there is no clear underlying cause, although dehydration, especially in the summer, is a factor. To reduce the risk of kidney stones it is important to drink at least 2 litres (3½ pints) of water each day and limit your intake of tea, coffee and alcohol.

Marine Life Injuries

What They Are

Not many marine creatures around Britain's shores pose a threat to bathers. The few dangerous sharks, such as the mako, sighted occasionally in coastal waters here have never been known to attack humans. But as climate change pushes up sea water temperatures, sharks and other tropical creatures will become more frequent visitors. Currently, the main risk to bathers (apart from drowning) comes from jellyfish, Portuguese man-o'-war and (rarely) weever fish, which give painful stings. People with pre-existing cardiac and respiratory conditions or allergies can suffer serious reactions to the toxins released. Pinch wounds from crabs and lobsters and scratches, scrapes and punctures from contact with coral, sea anemone or sea urchin tentacles are usually minor irritants. However, when untreated they can cause nasty infections.

Abroad, however, especially in the waters around the USA, Australia and South Africa, swimmers can incur a wide range of life-threatening injuries from all sorts of marine life. For example, shark, alligator, crocodile and moray eel bites can tear through skin, crush and break or sever bones. Sea snake venom has more than double the toxicity of cobra venom and a sea wasp (jellyfish) sting can kill a healthy patient in 15 minutes.

What to Look for

- Pain, red-hot rash, muscle cramps, stomach pain, fever, chills, nausea, vomiting, laboured breathing and collapse (severe sting reactions, also known as anaphylaxis).

- Laboured or difficult breathing.
- Cold, clammy skin or sluggishness.
- Joint pain and swelling.
- Spines or tentacles.
- Bleeding.
- Broken, crushed or severed bones.
- Open puncture wounds, cuts, scratches and scrapes.

What to Do

- Remove the patient from the water.
- Check whether the patient is breathing or has a pulse. If not, call 999 immediately and start CPR at once (see page 192).
- Stop bleeding by applying gentle pressure on the wound with a clean cloth until the bleeding stops (see page 201).
- If the patient seems to be in shock (cold, clammy skin or sluggishness), elevate his/her feet and keep the patient warm and comfortable.
- Immobilize broken bones (see page 203).
- If possible, find out what kind of marine life caused the injury in order to assure that the patient gets the proper treatment.
- Cleanse closed wounds with antiseptic soap or sea water.
- Loosely bandage or apply sterile gauze pads to open wounds.
- Remove spines or tentacles left by marine creatures with tweezers. Soak the wound in hot (not scalding) water until the pain eases, and elevate the patient's feet.
- Apply ice packs or a thick mix of bicarbonate of soda (baking soda) to ease pain.
- For sea snake bites follow the instructions for snake bites on page 43.

What Not to Do

- Don't move the patient's head or neck if he/she is unconscious.
- Don't apply alcohol, suntan oil or vinegar as this may cause more stings to discharge.
- Don't cut open a sea snake bite or sea wasp sting and try to suck out venom.

Typical Treatment

Large wounds will usually be cleaned and dead skin and foreign substances will be removed. Although large wounds are stitched, small wounds are usually left open, irrigated and covered with sterile dressing. Patients receive tetanus injections if they have not been immunized in the previous five years. They will also be evaluated to see if they need minor surgery and/or antibiotics. The pain and discomfort from most sea stings is of short duration. However, when burning, itching and warmness persist, the patient will be given topical antibiotics and tetanus toxoid injections. In the most serious cases of allergic reactions (anaphylaxis), intravenous adrenaline injections will be given.

After-care

Wounds usually close without the need for stitching. They should be examined every two to three days to monitor the healing process and check for infection.

Doctor Says

We have always had an ambivalent relationship with the creatures of deep – and shallow – waters. Always be aware of the possible dangers whenever you enter their realm!

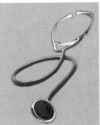

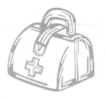

Neck Injuries

What They Are

The spinal cord is a long column of delicate nerves that connects the brain to receptors, muscles and organs throughout the body. Thirty-three bones called vertebrae protect the spinal cord. They sit one on top of another and are connected by ligaments and separated by discs. In addition to protecting the spinal cord, the vertebrae support the chest and abdomen. As the spinal cord ascends towards the skull, it becomes more complex because it is joined by increasing numbers of nerves, first from the legs, then the pelvis, abdomen, chest and arms.

Injuries occur when the cervical spine, the seven vertebrae of the neck, is forced into twisted, over-flexed, over-extended or other unnatural positions. Bones may fracture or dislocate and pinch, compress or sever spinal nerves, which can cause severe pain, irreversible nerve damage and paralysis. However, cervical spine injuries don't necessarily produce immediate or permanent damage.

Osteoarthritis can involve the bones of the neck. Slipped disks in the cervical neck area are rare.

Because of the complexity of the cervical spine, neck injuries may cause more severe nerve damage than lower spinal injuries. Furthermore, since the portion of the spine that supports the chest and abdomen is more rigid, trauma to the body is often transmitted to the flexible vertebrae in the neck. As a result, patients injured in car accidents often have 'whiplash' injuries to the neck.

Patients with severe osteoporosis or bone cancer can suffer major injuries from relatively minor trauma. In the direst cases, cervical spine injuries can paralyse both arms, both legs and the diaphragm and prevent patients from moving or breathing.

Car accidents, sports injuries, falls and other trauma can also injure soft tissue structures (muscles, ligaments, tendons) and internal organs (windpipe, digestive tract, thyroid) of the neck.

Patients may feel stiffness and pain caused by swelling or bleeding in the neck muscles but appear normal to observers.

Bullet and knife wounds to the neck are extremely dangerous because they usually involve highly critical organs that are close to the surface. Stabbing and gunshot victims will need surgery once their heart and circulation have stabilized.

What to Look for

- Neck pain, tenderness or stiffness, which is often felt hours later.
- Back, arm or leg pain or stiffness.
- Paralysis of the arms, legs or shoulders. Inability to move the toes.
- Numbness, tingling or no feeling in the arms, legs or shoulders.
- Shortness of breath (if the diaphragm or windpipe is affected).
- Nausea and vomiting.
- Hoarseness, difficulty swallowing, 'laryngitis'-type speech (indicates damage to internal structures of the neck).

What to Do

- Call 999 immediately so that emergency medical personnel can evaluate, stabilize and transport the patient.
- After calling 999, keep the patient's neck and other affected areas motionless, even if

the patient claims to be okay. *Immobilization is the highest priority!* Since it is possible for people to walk with unstable spine fractures, don't allow patients to move.

- Support the patient's spine with small pieces of wood, heavy towels, sandbags or a cervical collar, if available. Never move a patient's neck in order to support it or move a twisted neck into the 'correct position'.
- Keep the patient lying flat. Patients with neck fractures may have very low blood pressure. If patients feel as if they're going to vomit, turn them and all supportive neck bracing to the side as a unit. This is sometimes called 'log rolling' and requires at least two people working in close coordination. Failure to turn the patient may result in the patient choking on vomit, which can be fatal.
- Check the patient's rate and depth of breathing. Neck injuries can paralyse the diaphragm, the muscle that facilitates breathing and CPR may be needed (see page 192).

What Not to Do
- Don't move a patient's neck in order to support it.
- Don't move, lift or transport a neck or spinal injury patient by yourself.
- Don't allow a neck or spinal injury patient to stand or walk.

Typical Treatment
Emergency medical personnel will strap the patient to a transport board to protect against further injury. At the hospital, X-rays will be taken of all seven neck vertebrae and other injured areas. Neurological examinations will be performed to look for spinal cord injuries that the initial X-rays might have missed. CT scans or MRI may also be necessary to check that supportive structures have not been damaged.

In the hospital, the patient will be monitored for at least 24 hours even if tests fail to show fractures or spinal cord damage. If X-rays reveal fractures, traction devices will keep the bones from pressing on the spinal cord nerves.

Seriously injured patients will be admitted to a surgical intensive care unit and examined by orthopaedic surgeons and neurosurgeons. If surgery is required, it may not be scheduled until after the patient's condition has stabilized, which usually takes several days. After surgery, patients will recuperate in a rehabilitation centre for spinal-cord-injury patients.

Blood pressure may plummet due to neck fractures (spinal shock). This will be relieved by slightly elevating the foot of the patient's bed. The patient's stomach will be emptied so the patient doesn't vomit and choke while lying on his back.

After-care

Patients who did not sustain fractures or dislocations should expect to experience considerable pain and stiffness for several days. Those who received soft-tissue injuries will be given soft cervical collars for neck support. Ice packs applied during the first 24 hours may reduce tissue swelling.

Patients should be re-examined by an orthopaedic surgeon about two or three days after discharge and, if full recovery isn't evident, about a week later. Mild muscle relaxants (methocarbamol) or anti-inflammatory medications (ibuprofen) may help ease the pain.

Doctor Says

Because the risk of permanent damage is so great, anyone remotely suspected of a vertebral fracture should be assumed to have one until hospital testing is completed. Follow the A&E adage: 'A person who has neck pain after being touched by a feather has a cervical spine fracture until proved otherwise.'

Nosebleeds

What They Are

Nosebleeds occur when blood vessels in the nasal passages get ruptured. They can occur without warning and be triggered by allergies, pollution, nose picking, overuse of nasal sprays, cold/dry weather, low humidity and, of course, a punch in the nose. When arteries deep inside the nose break, often from hypertension and arteriosclerosis, blood can drain down the back of the throat and may not be outwardly visible.

Patients who suffer from impaired blood clotting (haemophilia and other related blood diseases) are susceptible to nosebleeds. People who take regular blood thinners, such as aspirin or warfarin, are also at risk. Offending medications may need to be discontinued, especially when arteries deep in the nasal cavity are damaged.

Since nosebleeds are common and usually stop within minutes, it is easy to minimize their significance. However, the blood loss from seemingly innocent nosebleeds can endanger elderly patients with poor circulation and heart problems. Persistent bleeding may cause them to choke on blood inhaled into their lungs.

What to Look for

- Bleeding from one nostril. Bleeding from both nostrils indicates a haemorrhage at the back of the nasal passages, an area that is inaccessible to pressure and cauterization.
- Pale, cold and clammy skin signifying blood loss.
- Blood draining down the back of the throat, a dangerous sign.

What to Do

- If the bleeding is from both nostrils, call 999 immediately.
- If the bleeding is from one nostril, check for blood in the throat, which indicates deep, internal nasal bleeding.
- If the bleeding is internal, call 999 immediately. Internal nosebleeds cannot be treated at home or in the GP's surgery.
- Keep the patient seated, head forward and facing downward, until arrival at a hospital.
- When the bleeding is from the front of the nose, apply cold compresses such as ice packs across the bridge of the nose that cover both sides.
- Pinch the nose for at least 10–15 minutes (as if there is a really bad smell).
- Allow the patient to sit slightly forward; never let the patient lie flat on his/her back.
- Get the patient to a hospital as soon as possible.

What Not to Do

- Don't let nosebleed patients touch or blow their noses. This could dislodge clots that are sealing leaking blood vessels.
- Don't pack nostrils with cotton wool. It could cause blood to accumulate and flow down the throat.
- Don't let a nosebleed patient lie on his/her back since he/she could choke on blood.

Typical Treatment

First, medical personnel will check the patient's vital signs. Serious blood loss can lower blood pressure and accelerate the pulse rate. Patients with abnormal vital signs due to blood loss should be hospitalized for observation for 24 hours.

The bleeding area, if visible, will be inspected with specialized lamps, mirrors and cauterizing tools. In most cases, the bleeding will have stopped and small scabs will be visible. Silver nitrate will be applied to control the bleeding. Adrenaline may be sprayed or swabbed onto the area to constrict bleeding vessels. If bleeding continues, surgical dressings will be packed into the nostril to compress the injured vessel. Packing should remain in place for two to three days.

Bleeding from deep in the nasal passages requires hospitalization. This type of bleeding is usually more profuse and the damaged blood vessels are usually hard to see and cauterize. To seal bleeding vessels, medical personnel will pack the nose, often using special nasal catheters (rubber tubes with small inflatable balloon tips filled with water). Catheters should remain in the nostrils until bleeding stops and patients' vital signs return to normal, which usually takes several days.

To prevent infection, patients will be given antibiotics. Laboratory tests will monitor clotting time, platelet count and assess the extent of the blood loss.

After-care

After two or three days, nasal packing is usually removed and further treatment is not required. Surgical repair (cauterization) of a nasal artery is rarely needed.

Patients should obtain information about medical and environmental conditions that might be causing their nosebleeds and address them. These can include high blood pressure, anticoagulant medication, dust or smog.

Doctor Says

Never underestimate nosebleeds and always err on the side of caution. Nosebleeds can be fatal. I once saw an otherwise healthy man die from nosebleed complications and a woman lose consciousness when her blood pressure dropped sharply. So, be on guard!

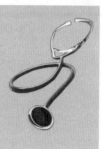

Paediatric Emergencies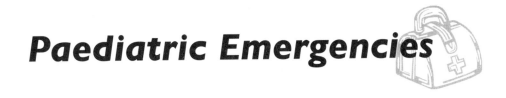

What They Are

Children can suffer virtually every type of medical emergency and diagnosis can be difficult because infants and small children can't describe what ails them. Paediatric emergencies can also be complicated by emotional factors such as fear, shyness and lack of control. In addition, a particular symptom may not indicate the actual problem and the child may simply be lethargic, irritable or not hungry.

Therefore, when you notice behavioural changes, fever, rash or pain, notify the family GP immediately. Medical staff in A&E units handle over 30 million paediatric cases each year, so erring on the side of caution is always advisable.

What to Look for

Intestinal Colic

- Children under six months old.
- Episodes of crying for several hours. The infant may be suffering from too much air in the intestines, hunger or dehydration.

Apnoea

- No breathing.
- Unresponsiveness.
- Turning blue.

Infectious Mononucleosis (glandula fever or the 'kissing disease')
- Red, sore throat and difficulty swallowing. May resemble a 'normal' sore throat.
- Swollen lymph nodes ('glands') in the neck.
- Yellow skin colour (jaundice), abdominal pain and nausea may indicate enlargement of the spleen or liver inflammation (hepatitis).

Sickle Cell Disease
- Severe pain anywhere in the body, but usually in the abdomen or limbs. Blood clots may form in small arteries, usually triggered by infection, dehydration or stress.
- Prevalent in those of Afro-Caribbean origin, usually in an inactive form (sickle-cell trait).

Skin Rash Due to Infectious Diseases
- Red, pink or white spots.
  - Measles: red spots first appear behind the ears.
  - Rubella: red spots first appear on face and neck.
  - Chickenpox: clear spots first appear on the trunk.
- Yellow bumps filled with pus, scaling and crusting of the lips, face and limbs are signs of impetigo, which is highly contagious.

Epiglottitis/Croup
- Swelling and narrowing of the upper airways.
- Difficulty breathing due to airflow obstruction.
- A high-pitched noise or wheeze when inhaling (stridor).
- Fever.
- 'Scratchy' voice.
- Difficulty swallowing.

- Coughing or drooling.

NOTE: Choking on objects (food or toys) has similar signs, except for fever.

Abdominal Pain
- A severe, diffuse, continuous abdominal pain that worsens with movement may indicate ruptured appendicitis and peritonitis.
- Pain occurring and disappearing in waves may be due to structural or mechanical abnormalities of the intestines, such as telescoping (intussusception), twisting (volvulus) or herniation (into the groin or umbilicus).

Febrile Seizures
- Rapid elevation of temperature.
- Sudden shaking of the entire body.
- Return to normal level of consciousness (unlike epilepsy).

Bronchiolitis
- Severe difficulty breathing.
- Wheezing (bronchiolitis may be a precursor to asthma).
- Runny nose.

Meningitis
- Fever and listlessness.
- Poor appetite, nausea and vomiting.
- Sensitivity to bright light.
- Neck stiffness.
- Possible seizures.

What to Do

Infants or children with any of the above conditions need immediate medical attention. If you suspect intestinal colic, mononucleosis or if the child has a rash, contact your GP. Otherwise:

- Call 999 immediately.
- Comfort and carefully watch the child.
- Perform CPR if the child stops breathing (see page 192).
- Perform abdominal thrusts (Heimlich manoeuvre) if the child is choking.

Intestinal Colic

Burp and comfort the infant, but it may not bring relief. When in doubt, call your GP.

Apnoea

Call 999 immediately and begin CPR to restore the child's circulation.

Infectious Mononucleosis

Call your GP. Give the child bed rest and fluids and keep the child away from other children. Expect two or more weeks for recovery.

Sickle Cell Disease

Call 999 immediately. A sickle cell crisis cannot be treated at home and requires inpatient hospital care.

Skin Rash: measles, rubella and chickenpox

Call your GP, who may suggest that you give the child Calpol (children's painkiller) and fluids.

Impetigo

Call your GP, who may prescribe antibiotics. Carefully cleanse the skin.

Epiglottitis/Croup

Call 999 immediately. The child will need hospital treatment to open constricted air passageways.

Perforated Appendicitis

Call 999 immediately, because the patient will require prompt surgery.

Febrile Seizures

Call 999 immediately. A&E evaluation is needed to ascertain the cause of the fever and to make sure that the child does not have epilepsy or meningitis. Stay calm – children snap out of febrile seizures once their temperatures go down.

Bronchiolitis

Call 999 immediately. Emergency medical personnel will give the child oxygen and may start intravenous fluids.

Meningitis

Call 999 immediately. Emergency personnel will give the child oxygen and may start intravenous fluids.

What Not to Do

- Don't give food or water to children who have abdominal pain, signs of meningitis, or breathing difficulties.

- Don't give children Calpol except on medical advice – it may mask symptoms and make diagnosis more difficult. Never give aspirin to children under 12 except on your GP's advice.

Typical Treatment

Intestinal Colic

There is no known medical treatment for this condition and it may need to be distinguished from life-threatening abdominal emergencies by your GP or A&E staff.

Apnoea

A&E staff will monitor and usually hospitalize all infants and children whose breathing may have stopped. It may then be necessary to carry out blood tests, X-rays, ECGs and other diagnostic tests.

Infectious Mononucleosis

There is no antibiotic treatment for this viral illness and recuperation may take several weeks. Patients will be monitored for signs of complications such as hepatitis and rupture of the spleen.

Sickle Cell Disease

Treatment may include pain medication, oxygen, intravenous fluids and possibly transfusions. A blood test can identify this genetic disease.

Skin Rash

After a few days of bed rest, measles, rubella and chickenpox usually pass without complications. Patients with impetigo will be given oral antibiotics.

Paediatric Emergencies

Epiglottitis/Croup

A&E staff will provide oxygen, adrenaline, intravenous corticosteroids and possibly antibiotics. Children who become lethargic or unable to breathe effectively may need mechanical ventilation or a tracheotomy. Choking on foreign objects can resemble epiglottitis or croup. If present, small inhaled items (beans, eraser tips, peas) may have to be removed under general anaesthesia.

Perforated Appendicitis

Immediate surgery is needed when appendicitis is complicated by peritonitis.

Febrile Seizures

A&E staff must locate the site of infection and may need to extract spinal fluid. Unlike epilepsy, there is no disorientation or confusion after the seizure. Treatment of the cause of fever (with Calpol and/or antibiotics) is of prime importance. Antiepilepsy medication is usually not needed. Children usually suffer no damage and outgrow this condition.

Bronchiolitis

Medication is given to open narrowed lung passages and patients will also receive oxygen, paracetamol and intravenous fluids. In severe cases, hospitalization and/or mechanical ventilation may be necessary.

Meningitis

A&E evaluation is needed immediately. Meningitis is a major medical emergency and patients will need intravenous antibiotics as soon as possible. Children who have been exposed to meningitis will need immediate medical evaluation and will usually be given oral antibiotics as a precautionary measure.

After-care

Children are amazingly resilient and most recover from paediatric emergencies without permanent complications or developmental problems. However, all patients should see their GP or a paediatrician several days after they were treated in A&E or hospitalized.

Make sure that children sleep on their back and not their tummy. Sleeping on the tummy is a risk factor for Sudden Infant Death Syndrome, a mysterious and poorly understood calamity of sudden respiratory arrest. Make sure an infant is warm but not too hot. If you have an infant or small child at home, don't allow visitors to smoke anywhere indoors – and certainly nowhere near the child.

Doctor Says

No one goes through childhood without several, hopefully minor, medical emergencies. Regular paediatric check-ups and good communication between parents and doctors decrease the possibility of serious problems and complications.

As a child, I contracted scarlet fever, a bacterial infection that resembles tonsillitis. My doctor recognized the raised red rash all over my body and my bright, strawberry-red tongue and gave me penicillin, which is still the accepted treatment for scarlet fever.

Phlebitis

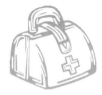

What It Is

Phlebitis is a condition in which blood clots (thrombi) form inside blood vessels. Although these clots can form in any blood vessel, they appear most commonly in the veins of women's legs. Phlebitis strikes pregnant women, women on oral contraceptives, bedridden and postoperative patients, as well as the obese, smokers, the elderly and those with varicose veins. Large blood clots can also block the arteries of patients with severe 'hardening of the arteries' and atrial fibrillation. Patients develop sudden pain in an arm or leg, which becomes pale, cold, numb or paralysed.

Phlebitis can be excruciatingly painful. However, superficial phlebitis, which affects veins visible on the leg's surface, is usually not life-threatening. When phlebitis is deep in hidden calf veins, it can be dangerous. Small pieces of a clot can break off, enter the bloodstream and block tiny arteries in the lungs. This can cut off circulation, injure the lung and block the normal exchange of oxygen and carbon dioxide (acute pulmonary embolism).

What To Look For

- Redness, swelling, warmth and tenderness in the affected area. Inflamed veins may appear near the surface of the leg.
- A pale, cold, numb or paralysed limb (acute arterial occlusion due to atrial fibrillation).
- Severe pain and swelling in the back of the lower leg, which often intensifies when standing or walking.

- Calf pain when moving the foot of the affected leg up and down.
- If patients with calf pain were recently confined to bed rest or were seated for prolonged periods (in aeroplanes, for example), assume that they might have phlebitis.
- Sudden shortness of breath, palpitations, chest pains and heart rhythm disturbances (acute pulmonary embolism).
- You may not be able to see or feel a clotted varicose vein.

What to Do

- Place the patient flat on his/her back.
- Elevate the leg until the affected vein is higher than the heart, unless the leg is pale, cold and numb.
- Place a warm compress on the inflamed, tender area, for example, a towel moistened with warm tap water.
- If the pain is severe call 999 and/or notify the patient's doctor.

What Not to Do

Do not allow patients to sit, stand or walk.

Typical Treatment

Blood tests, ECGs or X-rays cannot confirm whether the patient has phlebitis. Therefore, the diagnosis is made primarily from the patient's history and from a physical examination. However, a Doppler ultrasound scan is often helpful.

Anticoagulants such as low-molecular weight heparin can be injected into the skin to thin the blood, inhibit clot growth and prevent clot fragments from travelling to the lungs. Usually, warfarin, an oral anticoagulant, is given – sometimes along with heparin – for the first two to three days (not suitable during the first three months of a pregnancy).

Patients receiving the stronger anticoagulants (for deep phlebitis) must be monitored for possible haemorrhaging unrelated to phlebitis, including bleeding stomach ulcers or blood in the urine.

Thanks to the body's natural anticoagulation process, blockages usually improve in about six to eight hours and clots in lung arteries (pulmonary emboli) become less likely.

After-care

Hospitalization usually lasts for several days as swelling, pain and redness disappear. After discharge, patients will remain on oral anticoagulants for several months to prevent further clotting. Elastic stockings that gently support the calf muscles also help the circulation, but other tight, constricting leg wear can be dangerous. Conditions that contribute to phlebitis such as inactivity, obesity and use of oral contraceptives must also be addressed.

Doctor Says

Proceed gently when elevating a patient's leg above the heart or when moving the patient's leg in any other way. Never squeeze or touch the affected area because you might cause a clot, or a piece of a clot, to break free and travel to the patient's lungs!

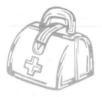

Pneumonia

What It Is

When infectious agents such as bacteria and viruses are inhaled, they can overwhelm the lungs' defence mechanisms and flood the lungs with secretions. This impairs the exchange of oxygen and carbon dioxide and causes shortness of breath, extreme weakness and sometimes delirium.

Pneumonia is one of the leading causes of death in the UK. The infection may be more severe for patients who are confined to nursing homes, as well as those suffering from emphysema, diabetes, chronic alcoholism or receiving chemotherapy for cancer.

'Walking pneumonia' is the condition where patients with pneumonia don't exhibit signs or symptoms of the disease. Unrecognized and untreated lung infections can be life-threatening.

Pleurisy is inflammation or infection of the membranes that line the lungs and it can be fatal. When severe, pleurisy can limit the lungs' ability to expand and inflate. This may allow bacteria to enter the bloodstream where they multiply and release toxins into the blood (septicaemia) that can cause a dangerous drop in the patient's blood pressure.

Acute bronchitis is a milder infection than pneumonia and is usually confined to the upper airways, not the lungs. Patients will have fever, muscle aches and runny nose, but none of the more dramatic symptoms.

What to Look for

- Shortness of breath.
- Rapid breathing. A pulse over 120 indicates a severe emergency.
- Severe coughing.
- Gurgling sounds when breathing.
- Green, yellow, bloody or 'rusty-coloured' phlegm.
- Muscle and joint pain.
- Severe fatigue, weakness or dizziness.
- Fever.
- Chills (uncontrollable shaking).
- Blue lips or fingertips.
- Appetite loss.
- Delirium or confusion.
- Pneumonia may have no clear-cut respiratory signs. So look for uncharacteristic irritability and restlessness in the very young and loss of appetite in the elderly.

What to Do

- Call 999 immediately if the patient appears dehydrated, disoriented, extremely weak or unable to drink.
- Take the patient for emergency treatment if he/she is breathing rapidly (more than 20 breaths per minute), making 'gurgling' sounds, has blue lips or fingertips, a severe cough or uncontrollable chills.
- Notify your GP, if possible. Pneumonia can be diagnosed in the GP's surgery, but patients who appear very ill may need A&E evaluation.
- Keep the patient warm, at rest and seated if possible (to avoid choking).
- Apply warm, moist compresses to the chest.

- Give the patient ibuprofen, aspirin or supplemental oxygen, if available.
- For bronchitis, call the patient's doctor and follow the instructions given.

What Not to Do

- Don't allow the patient to minimize his/her condition by suggesting, 'It's only flu.'
- Don't let the patient use other people's antibiotics, because they may undermine laboratory tests.

Typical Treatment

A chest X-ray will usually reveal the presence of pneumonia. Blood tests will determine the severity of the infection and degree of respiratory impairment. Oxygen and intravenous fluids are administered to stabilize the patient's vital signs and circulation.

When tests identify offending bacteria (viruses cannot be cultured or seen under the usual microscopes), antibiotics are given. Antibiotics will be started as soon as bacteria coughed up in a sputum sample have been identified under a microscope.

When infections are life-threatening, two intravenous antibiotics are immediately given to prevent septicaemia. They are often started before the test results are available.

Although hospital confinement is usually preferred for seriously ill patients, A&E staff will decide whether to admit a patient or send him/her home with oral antibiotics. Medications prescribed include penicillin, erythromycin and doxycycline.

A patient with pneumonia that affects both lungs or that produces large amounts of respiratory secretions is monitored in the intensive care unit. Bed rest and a nutritious diet (either at home or in the hospital) are required for the patient's recovery.

After-care

Expect it to take at least a week for signs of recovery to occur. Full recovery can take longer with patients who also suffer from conditions such as diabetes, emphysema, cystic fibrosis, asthma and coronary disease. A patient should continue taking antibiotics until the fever, white cell count, high respiratory rate and cough are under control.

Doctor Says

Practise counting respiration rates so that you can tell if a patient's breathing is impaired. Watch and count the chest expansions of your family and friends. The normal rate is 18 breaths per minute. If you suspect pneumonia, look for shaking chills – the most ominous sign of the condition – and, if they are present, get emergency help!

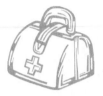

Poisoning and Drug Abuse

What They Are

Adverse physical or mental reactions can occur when we ingest, inhale or touch toxic substances – solid, liquid or gas. These toxins can destroy organs, cells and tissues and prevent our systems from functioning properly. The damage can be immediate, delayed or both and may or may not have characteristic signs or symptoms.

Antidotes exist for some poisons, but not all. In the absence of antidotes, critically ill patients will be connected to machines that breathe for them (mechanical ventilators) and monitored in an intensive care unit until the poison is metabolized, neutralized and excreted.

Carbon monoxide, cocaine and tricyclic antidepressants are the most deadly of toxic substances. They are then followed by paracetamol, tranquillizers, lead and opiates (primarily heroin).

Recreational drugs can be lethal, especially when several drugs are taken together – for example, alcohol, sedatives and stimulants. Only hospitals are equipped to handle these complex emergencies.

Other medical emergencies caused by specific poisons include seizures, heart-rhythm disturbances, breathing disorders, coma, hyperthermia (extremely high body temperature) and blood-chemistry imbalances. Since dangerous chemicals remain in the bloodstream for hours, patients can develop any of these life-threatening conditions when the toxins are in their systems.

What to Look for

- Incoherent speech.
- Small pupils or extremely wide pupils.
- Blue lips or fingertips.
- Stumbling while walking.
- Shallow breathing.
- Disorientation.
- Seizures.
- Signs of an apparent suicide attempt.

What to Do

- For drug overdoses or severe poisonings, call 999 immediately. Time is of the essence – a life could be in danger!
- When in doubt, call 999 promptly. It is often impossible to know how much poison a patient has absorbed. So, always err on the side of caution, because a patient's respiratory rate or blood pressure can drop suddenly.
- If a patient inhales and collapses from noxious chemicals (smoke or chemical emissions), remove the patient from exposure, if possible and safe to do so (but do not put yourself in danger).
- Call 999 immediately and try to provide fresh air until emergency medical personnel arrive. For example, move the patient into the open, if possible and safe to do so, or open windows to allow fresh air to enter the room.
- Use fresh water to carefully wash away any chemical that has been left on the patient's skin.
- Place the patient on one side until emergency personnel arrive to eliminate the danger of choking on vomit.

- If there are pills or bottles nearby that may be the cause of the poisoning, collect them and hand to emergency medical personnel as they may help to identify the poison responsible and so indicate the correct antidote.

What Not to Do

- Don't try to induce vomiting. There is no evidence that this reduces the amount of poison ingested and there is a major risk that the noxious substance may be inhaled into the lungs and/or may cause burning to the oesophagus.

Typical Treatment

Treatment will initially focus on stabilizing the patient's vital signs; cardiac monitoring and respiratory support. Poisonous substances will be neutralized, or may be removed, and intravenous fluids may be administered to normalize blood pressure and speed the metabolism of toxins.

The standard treatment in most cases of swallowed poisons is repeated administration of activated charcoal, especially when the cause of poisoning or an overdose is unknown. The activated charcoal binds potentially toxic chemicals before they pass from the intestines to the bloodstream. Sometimes the patient's stomach may be washed out, although this is no longer routine. Otherwise the medical priorities are supportive care (such as mechanical ventilation and monitoring in an intensive care unit) and treatment of symptoms as they arise. Chest X-rays may be arranged to check for accidental inhalation of stomach contents.

Antidotes exist for some poisons. For example, naloxone is the antidote for opiate intoxication. Naloxone immediately reverses heroin, morphine, codeine or methadone overdoses and may cause withdrawal, which in itself can be a medical emergency.

Other specific poison remedies include high doses of oxygen for carbon monoxide, dialysis for medications such as lithium or pH (acid–alkaline) imbalances, chelation for lead and mercury, sodium nitrite and sodium thiosulphate for cyanide, atropine for insecticide and diazepam for antidepressants. In the case of paracetamol poisoning, activated charcoal may be given for small doses ingested within the previous 12 hours. Otherwise acetylcysteine or methionine is given to protect the liver from damage.

Patients who took or were exposed to dangerous toxins that metabolize slowly will remain hospitalized, often in the intensive care unit, where they will be monitored and treated.

After-care

After patients are discharged from A&E, their family and friends should monitor their behaviour closely. Patients who overdosed on recreational drugs or as a result of suicide attempts will undergo psychological evaluation before they are discharged.

After discharge, they should continue counselling.

Doctor Says

Treat every poisoning and drug overdose as life-threatening. Don't delay calling 999. While you are waiting for help to arrive, place the patient on one side to prevent choking should vomiting occur.

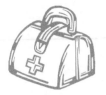

Seizures

What They Are

Seizures are uncontrollable, severe, spasmodic body movements (jerking) that are accompanied by altered levels of consciousness. Seizures are also known as epileptic seizures or convulsions. Epilepsy, a major cause of seizures, can be a hereditary condition that begins in childhood or adolescence and can last a lifetime. In some cases it follows head injury or infection.

Seizures fall into several classifications. Generalized seizures (grand mal epilepsy) are the most dramatic because patients lose consciousness, fall to the ground and their bodies shake with convulsions. Convulsions often alternate with the spastic extension of all four limbs. Seizure attacks usually last one to two minutes and are often followed by loss of bladder control.

During a seizure, a patient may bite the tongue, fracture or dislocate bones, or inhale vomit or respiratory secretions. Therefore, prompt emergency medical care should be sought, especially if the seizures are continuous or recur during a 30-minute period and the patient does not regain consciousness.

When a seizure ends, patients are usually in a stupor for 10–20 minutes, followed by 20–30 minutes of extreme confusion and disorientation.

Absence seizures (petit mal epilepsy) usually last only a few seconds. Patients typically stare blankly while their eyelids blink. They don't collapse or shake with convulsions. When they regain consciousness, they have no memory of the seizure.

Seizures

Partial seizures are due to abnormal electrical discharges in one area of the brain. Patients usually experience a specific physical reaction, principally twitching of a single body part such as one arm or leg. Partial and petit mal seizures are less life-threatening than generalized or grand mal seizures. However, after their initial episode, all patients should get emergency treatment as soon as possible.

Seizures occurring after a head injury are called secondary or post-traumatic epilepsy. Seizures can also be caused by high fever, sedative or alcohol withdrawal, sleep deprivation, stress or abuse of stimulants. See Obstetric Disorders on page 183 for a discussion of pre-eclampsia, a syndrome of high blood pressure and oedema that affects pregnant women and can lead to life-threatening seizures if untreated.

What to Look for
- Convulsions (erratic bodily jerking).
- Loss of consciousness.
- Stretching or extending all four limbs.
- Loss of bladder control.
- Confusion and disorientation.
- Flashing lights, strange smells, 'pins and needles' tingling that lasts 20–30 seconds (unusual premonitions called 'auras' are experienced by some patients).

What to Do
- Call 999, but don't leave a patient alone during a seizure, even to call 999. Make sure the patient's condition has stabilized before calling 999.
- Lay the patient down so that he/she can't fall.
- Turn the patient on his/her side to prevent choking on gastric or respiratory secretions (or blood, if the tongue is accidentally bitten).

What Not to Do

- Don't leave the patient unattended during a seizure, even to call 999.
- Don't allow the patient to fall.
- Don't push anything into the patient's mouth. It might push the patient's tongue further back and cause him/her to choke.

Typical Treatment

Hospitalization for 24-hour observation is usually needed for first-time sufferers. Patients who had seizures due to head injuries and pregnant woman with pre-eclampsia are always admitted for observation and treatment. Patients with chronic epilepsy may be discharged if they recover quickly and did not sustain any significant physical injuries.

A seizure patient receives intravenous medication such as diazepam or phenobarbital to stabilize his/her condition. Patients are given tests that aid in diagnosis including CT scans or MRI, electroencephalograms (EEGs) and lumbar punctures. Unfortunately, some test results may be deceptively normal between seizures.

After-care

The patient's doctor or consulting neurologist will decide whether to put the patient on daily antiepileptic medication such as carbamazepine or valproate (vaplroic acid). Although many antiepileptic drugs exist, they all have side effects. Medication taken regularly usually stops most seizures, but many patients on medication still have 'breakthrough' seizures. Social and psychological factors such as stress, fatigue, embarrassment and discrimination should be addressed. By understanding the nature of their condition and epilepsy itself, patients and their families can handle it more effectively.

Doctor Says

Many epileptics sense the onset of an attack. Despite the dramatic nature of epilepsy, seizures don't directly traumatize the brain or the body. Patients usually return to normal after about an hour of sleepiness and confusion.

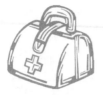

Skin Emergencies and Allergies

What They Are

When we come in contact with certain toxic substances, the skin acts as the body's first line of defence. It warns us of danger by breaking out in lesions, nettle rash (urticaria), bumps and blotches and by making us sniffle or itch and our eyes water. These signals are hard to ignore, but it is surprising how many people pay them no heed.

Rash and skin eruptions account for about 5 per cent of adult and 30 per cent of child A&E visits. Drug, food and other allergies are among the most common causes of skin emergencies. Often, they are the first warning to steer clear of shellfish, peanuts, penicillin, cats, wool and other irritants. Other substances that trigger allergic reactions include aspirin, milk, eggs, sulfa drugs, nickel (in jewellery and watch-straps), iodine contrast dyes, mismatched blood transfusions and wasp, bee and ant stings. When sensitive patients come in contact with these items, they can get severe allergic reactions that, if not promptly treated, can be life-threatening.

Shingles is a reactivation of chickenpox virus in adults that affects the nerves of the trunk, face or eye, usually on one side only. Shingles produces an extremely painful rash but is not contagious.

Sunburn is a painful superficial burn caused by prolonged exposure to ultraviolet light (see Burns on page 54).

What to Look for

- Bumps on the skin, either clear nettle rash (urticaria) or reddened rash.
- Complaints that 'my entire body is hot' or 'itchy'.
- Swelling of the face, neck or tongue.
- Rash or other lesions in the mouth may warn of impending upper airway constriction. Additional signs are patients sounding hoarse, coughing and developing shortness of breath.
- Ask:
  - Where is the rash? Is it localized to one part of the body or everywhere?
  - Did it occur suddenly or gradually?
  - Does it hurt, itch or neither?
  - Did it become apparent after exposure or contact with food, drugs or plants?
  - Did the rash appear after exposure to sunlight?
  - What colour is the rash?
  - How old is the patient? (To rule out measles or chickenpox.)
  - Is the patient taking prescription medication?
- Skin lesions all over the body could indicate dangerous infectious diseases such as meningitis.
- A small, itchy rash on a single body part usually indicates a localized allergic reaction (contact dermatitis) that was activated by touching an irritant such as fabrics, plants, jewellery, hair products or cosmetics.
- Extremely painful clusters of 'bubbles' on one side of the torso or face may be shingles.
- Redness, blistering and pain after prolonged exposure to the sun is in most cases sunburn.

What to Do

- Call 999 immediately if the patient has swelling or rash in the mouth. Speed is of the essence since the patient's breathing passages could constrict.
- Call 999 if the patient has swelling of the face, neck, lips or tongue (angiodoema).
- Call 999 immediately if the patient sounds hoarse or is short of breath. The patient's blood pressure could plummet and the patient may collapse (anaphylactic shock).
- Call 999 immediately if the patient has a rash all over his/her body, fever, malaise, headache, vomiting or neck stiffness (meningitis).
- Rush a child with a rash to accident and emergency. Their problem could be relatively harmless (chickenpox or measles) or extremely serious (meningitis).

What Not to Do

- Don't allow the patient to downplay symptoms, especially if you see the rash worsen.
- Don't attempt to diagnose a child's condition. Just rush him/her to A&E.

Typical Treatment

A small, itchy rash due to localized allergic reactions is usually treated with over-the-counter corticosteroid creams. Superficial infections and abscesses generally respond to topical (applied) or oral antibiotics or draining. Infection of deeper tissue layers (cellulitis) is normally treated with intravenous antibiotics and may require hospitalization.

Emergency facilities treat allergic reactions with antihistamines and injections of adrenaline-like medication. A patient suspected of having upper airway obstruction may be hospitalized because, even if he/she initially improves, potentially fatal toxins may remain in the bloodstream. The most serious cases may be given intravenous adrenaline, antihistamines or corticosteroids, and receive mechanical support for breathing.

For shingles, acyclovir pills are prescribed for one week.

WARNING: If you treat an allergic reaction at home with antihistamines, follow up with a phone call to your GP, asking him/her to examine the patient as soon as possible.

After-care

Patients will be discharged from A&E when their intense initial itching, warmness and redness begin to subside, which usually takes three to four hours. They should continue taking antihistamines for another day or two.

A skin rash can last for at least a week, long after the toxic trigger has left the body. Patients should be reassured that his/her appearance won't be affected since cosmetic damage seldom occurs.

Doctor Says

Second or subsequent reactions often increase in intensity and can result in a catastrophic drop of blood pressure (anaphylactic shock). If you have had an allergic reaction, find out what caused it and eliminate it from your life. Keep suitable antihistamine tablets at home (ask your pharmacist for advice). They can be obtained without prescription. Ask your doctor whether an emergency kit containing injectable adrenaline would be advisable in your case.

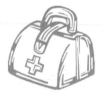

Stroke

What Is It

Stroke is one of the leading causes of death in the UK: more than 40,000 deaths occur annually. Stroke is also a major cause of disability: it can paralyse patients permanently and may mean that they are left unable to care for themselves. Stroke is caused by blood clots (thrombi) or large pieces of cholesterol plaque that block arteries and cut off the circulation of oxygen to the brain. When nerve cells are deprived of oxygen, they die in a few minutes.

Emboli (pieces of blood clots) cause blockages when they travel downstream from either the heart walls or the inner surface of the large carotid arteries in the neck.

Extremely high blood pressure, usually 220/120 or more, may cause blood vessels to break and bleed directly into brain tissue (haemorrhagic stroke).

Aneurysms are small weak areas in the cerebral arterial walls that may swell, burst and flood the brain with blood.

A stroke affecting the breathing centre of the brain can cause a heart attack and, conversely, stroke can be triggered by heart attacks.

TIA (transient ischaemic attack) is a temporary neurological impairment that is caused by a blocked cerebral artery. If it is not immediately treated, it can cause permanent damage. TIAs last less than 24 hours and about 80 per cent of cases tend to be resolved within 30 minutes.

What to Look for

- Inability to move, stand, talk or communicate. A patient may be unable to answer simple questions or identify family members.
- Paralysis. Usually, only one side of the body and specific functions are affected. For example, a patient with a clot on the left side of the brain (which affects the speech and motor areas) cannot move the right side of his/her body and cannot talk.
- Severe headache.
- Double vision.
- Dizziness.
- Nausea and vomiting.

What to Do

- Call 999 immediately. Prompt action can truly be a matter of life or death.
- Call 999 immediately if the patient is a diabetic. Hypoglycaemia due to an insulin reaction may look exactly like a stroke.
- Check whether the patient is breathing and has a pulse. If not, begin CPR (see page 192).
- If a patient is nauseous or vomiting, tilt the head or body slightly to one side.
- Keep an alert patient resting comfortably because balance and ability to bear weight may be impaired.

What Not to Do

Don't give aspirin and similar pain relievers to patients with severe headache and nausea. Aspirin is a blood thinner that could exacerbate stroke caused by bleeding into the brain. Stronger painkillers may have a sedating effect on patients, which can also be dangerous.

Typical Treatment

Initially, emergency medical personnel will try to stabilize the patient's heart and breathing functions by giving oxygen, intravenous fluids and antihypertensive medication, when appropriate. When a patient is stabilized, CT scan will determine whether an area of the brain did not receive blood or blood has flooded and compressed brain tissue.

A patient having a stroke caused by the blockage of a narrow, arteriosclerotic artery may receive blood thinners, such as heparin, aspirin or alteplase (given within six hours of the stroke). Alteplase is an intravenous medication that helps dissolve clots and restore blood flow. However, a patient with documented bleeding into the brain cannot receive blood thinners. A consulting neurologist will decide which medications are appropriate.

ECGs will check for heart damage and rhythm disturbances. Chest X-rays may be taken to detect pneumonia. Echocardiograms may reveal clots on the inner surface of the heart (a potential source of emboli).

After-care

Patients, including those with TIAs, must continue to be hospitalized. The extent of their neurological damage will be assessed and their condition will be monitored. Other necessary tests may include carotid ultrasound scans and cerebral angiograms. Blockages found in neck arteries can sometimes be removed by a surgical procedure (carotid endarterectomy).

When the acute illness passes, physical rehabilitation and psychological support will begin, which can be a long, arduous road.

Patients who are unable to care for themselves must have full-time in-home care or be placed in nursing homes.

Doctor Says

Always check a suspected stroke patient's pulse and breathing. Stroke victims often run a high risk of other clot-related illnesses such as heart attacks. Place patients slightly to one side, not flat on their backs, so that they don't choke on gastric or respiratory secretions.

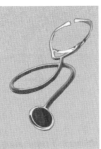

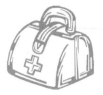

Urinary Tract Disorders

What They Are

Medical problems can occur along the path that urine travels after it forms in the kidneys. These problems can be infections or dysfunctions of the kidneys, the ureter (the tube that carries urine to the bladder), the bladder (the organ that stores urine until it is expelled) and the urethra (the opening through which urine exits the body).

Men may also suffer from swelling or infection of the prostate gland, a walnut-sized organ that can enlarge and compress the urethra. Untreated urinary tract infections may develop into life-threatening kidney infections.

Urine rarely contains harmful amounts of bacteria because of its acid chemistry. However, when the outflow is partially blocked by an enlarged prostate, a pregnancy or a kidney stone, bacteria can multiply in the stagnant urinary system. *Escherichia coli*, pathogens normally found in the large intestine, are the most common culprit. Women are more prone to urinary tract infections than men because their urethra is shorter and so more vulnerable to external bacteria.

Acute urinary retention occurs when the urinary path is suddenly blocked for some reason. Men over the age of 60 may get this painful condition when the prostate gland enlarges and therefore prevents the bladder from emptying properly. If urine and bacteria back up into the kidneys and/or the bloodstream (*urosepsis*), this can cause shock or even death.

What to Look for

Bladder Infections (cystitis)

- Burning sensation during urination.
- A dramatic increase in urinary frequency (often hourly).
- Pain in the central lower abdomen (the bladder area).
- Fever.
- Blood in the urine.

Kidney Infections (pyelonephritis)

- The symptoms listed above plus:
- Severe pain on one side of the lower back.
- Nausea, vomiting and shaking chills.

Urinary Retention

- Pain and swelling over the central lower abdomen (bladder).

What to Do

- When a urinary tract infection is suspected, call the patient's doctor immediately.
- When the patient has chills, vomiting and/or flank pain, immediately call 999.
- If urine is being retained (pain over the bladder), immediately call 999.

What Not to Do

- Don't delay calling 999 if urinary retention or acute kidney infections are even remotely suspected.
- Don't give a patient another person's antibiotics. Those medicines may be ineffective or harmful and may complicate proper diagnosis.

Typical Treatment

The patient's history, vital signs and physical examination will determine the severity of his/her condition. Blood and urine tests will confirm whether the patient has a bladder infection. A urine culture will be taken to identify the presence of specific bacteria and to determine which antibiotics are most effective. An extremely ill patient will have blood cultured to see if actively multiplying bacteria have entered the circulatory system. Antibiotics are often given before the results are available.

Emergency patients with acute urinary retention may need a bladder catheterization. In this procedure, a doctor inserts a thin, sterile, rubber tube into the urinary tract. The tube opens a pathway and allows urine to drain from the bladder. The urine expelled will be examined for signs of infection.

Patients with kidney infections, urinary blockage or sepsis (bacteria in the bloodstream) will usually be hospitalized and given intravenous fluids and antibiotics. Expect hospitalization to last for at least a week. Consultations with a urologist and diagnostic X-ray tests should determine the correct diagnosis and the appropriate course of treatment.

When a man under 50 years old has symptoms such as burning pain when urinating or during sex, it is usually due to a sexually transmitted disease such as gonorrhea or chlamydia. Treatment includes antibiotics including penicillin, amoxicillin, ceftriaxone and metronidazole. The patient's sexual partner is contacted and treated to prevent further spread of the disease.

After-care

Most patients with uncomplicated urinary tract infections receive oral antibiotics (nitrofurantoin, ciprofloxacin or methenamine hippurate) and are sent home. They should see their doctor a few days after A&E discharge. Patients should continue taking medication for three to ten days as directed by their doctor, at which time their urine will be re-examined and recultured to determine whether or not all infectious agents have disappeared.

Patients with more complex problems will continue to be monitored by their doctor.

Doctor Says

Urinary tract infections account for over six million visits to the GP every year, and two-thirds of the patients are women. Painful bladder infections account for the bulk of these visits. If you think that you are getting a bladder infection, drink lots of cranberry juice, monitor your condition and get help if your symptoms persist. When I developed sudden urinary retention after surgery about ten years ago, I thought that I would explode! My sympathies go to anyone who might have a similar experience.

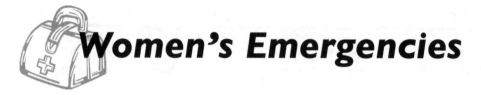

Women's Emergencies

Gynaecological Emergencies

What They Are

Women's emergencies usually fall into two basic categories: those involving pregnancy and those involving abnormal inflammation or bleeding of the reproductive organs. The early diagnosis of gynaecological emergencies can be difficult because of the complex anatomy involved and because so many of the symptoms are shared with those of other ailments.

Vaginal Bleeding

During normal menstruation, blood loss is between 30 and 60cc (requiring one to three tampons for absorption). Women may also experience a consistent pattern of mild cramping at certain points of the menstrual cycle over the course of their lives. Vaginal bleeding becomes a medical emergency when the volume of blood, the duration of the bleeding, the time of the month when bleeding occurs and other symptoms (cramping, vomiting, abdominal pain and clotting) differ from the patient's usual menstrual pattern. Since normal menstrual bleeding doesn't clot, heavy or rapid bleeding and the presence of clots may indicate abnormalities including fibroid tumours, hormonal imbalances or cancer of the uterus or cervix. Both birth control pills and hormone replacement therapy (HRT) can also cause abnormal or heavy bleeding. Post-menopausal bleeding always requires investigation.

Fibroid Tumours

About 25 per cent of women have fibroid tumours – abnormal muscle growths in the womb. After years of unnoticed enlargement, fibroid tumours can bleed excessively, but few haemorrhage enough to require urgent care. Gynaecologists can often feel fibroid tumours during pelvic examinations.

Ovarian Cysts

Abnormal ovulation can cause ovarian cysts, small growths on the surface of the ovary, that may swell and rupture. A bursting ovarian cyst immediately causes severe discomfort. In contrast, ovarian cancer grows slowly and silently, making detection difficult.

Ectopic (Tubal) Pregnancies

Abdominal or pelvic pain without vaginal bleeding can indicate an ectopic (tubal) pregnancy. An ectopic pregnancy occurs when a fertilized egg is implanted in a Fallopian tube, not in the uterine wall. The surrounding tissues can't support foetal development. Intense pain and nausea ensue. When the foetus dies and uterine bleeding is heavy, the patient's blood pressure may suddenly drop. Ectopic pregnancy occurs in about 2 per cent of all pregnancies. It is the most lethal gynaecological emergency because blood may enter and inflame the abdominal cavity.

Other causes of heavy menstrual bleeding and/or pelvic pain include:

- Benign polyps of the cervix or uterus – the excessive growth of normal tissue.
- Pelvic inflammatory disease (PID) of the female reproductive organs – is usually a sexually transmitted disease (gonorrhea or chlamydia) affecting the Fallopian tubes, uterus or an ovary. In serious cases it can form abscesses that rupture, leading to bacterial peritonitis.

- Endometriosis – the implanting of normal uterine tissue in abnormal areas of the pelvis or abdomen. Endometriosis is found in between 5 and 10 per cent of women and is thought to be the result of retrograde menstruation (menstruation that flows in the wrong direction). It causes cyclical discomfort that will be continuous if scarring occurs.

What to Look for

- Heavy or rapid vaginal bleeding.
- Sudden or severe pelvic or abdominal pain.
- Nausea, vomiting.
- Fever, vaginal discharge, lower abdominal pain (PID or pelvic abscess).
- Fatigue, nausea and loss of appetite (could indicate the spread of uterine or cervical cancer).
- Dizziness, light-headedness, anxiety or fainting (may be signs of unstable blood pressure).
- Shoulder pain may be due to blood that is causing inflammation of the inner abdominal membranes and the lower diaphragm surface (possibly indicating ectopic pregnancy).

What to Do

- Call 999 immediately.
- Have the patient rest comfortably, preferably lying down with her knees elevated to avoid dizziness, faintness or collapse.
- Gynaecological emergencies are always emotionally draining so patients will need both cardiovascular and psychological support.

What Not to Do

- Don't leave the patient unattended after calling 999.
- Don't allow the patient to eat, drink or take over-the-counter medications. For example, aspirin could thin the blood and worsen haemorrhaging and paracetamol could mask characteristic painful symptoms.
- Don't touch the abdomen. It could lead to nausea, vomiting or circulatory collapse if pressure causes an ovarian cyst, ectopic pregnancy or pelvic abscess to rupture.

Typical Treatment

Emergency medical personnel will assess the severity of the patient's condition by checking her vital signs. Their primary concern is stabilizing her blood pressure and tissue oxygenation.

Laboratory testing will determine if a patient is pregnant. If she has lost substantial amounts of blood she will be given intravenous fluids, nasal oxygen and perhaps transfusions. Her pelvic organs will be examined for signs of bleeding, infection, uterine fibroids, ovarian masses and cancer.

A patient with an ectopic pregnancy will receive immediate surgery if she has low blood pressure, a fast heart rate and a low blood count. Some younger patients may be candidates for limited surgery to remove only the affected portion of the Fallopian tube while others might be injected with methotrexate, which causes an ectopic abortion.

Often, a pelvic ultrasound scan can identify ectopic pregnancy, fibroid tumours, ovarian cysts/abscesses, endometriosis and some cancers. If found, a hysteroscopy (examination of the uterus using a fibre-optic camera) or a biopsy may be needed.

Women aged over 35 who have abnormal vaginal bleeding may be treated as outpatients if their vital signs and test results are normal.

Gynaecological emergencies not due to pregnancy must be evaluated for irritation or infection of the abdominal cavity (peritonitis). If blood has entered the abdomen, immediate exploratory surgery will be necessary.

Vaginal bleeding due to fibroid tumours, cancer or infection will be treated when the underlying condition is diagnosed.

PID is treated with oral or intravenous antibiotics. Severe cases are admitted for hospitalization to prevent complications such as ectopic pregnancy and infertility.

Many subtypes of menstrual bleeding respond to hormone therapy, birth control pills or anti-inflammatory medications such as ibuprofen and naproxen.

After-care

The length of hospitalization depends on the type of emergency and the extent of bleeding, infection or secondary complications including peritonitis. The patient should be examined by her GP or gynaecologist a few days after being discharged from the hospital.

Doctor Says

Regular gynaecological check-ups are essential. Often, they can prevent the onset of serious emergencies. Many PID cases are undiagnosed and can lead to ectopic pregnancies and infertility. Patients who suspect PID should get prompt treatment and counselling, as should their partners. Post-menopausal bleeding and abdominal pain during menstruation are always abnormal, so see your doctor immediately.

Obstetric Disorders

What They Are

During pregnancy, women can develop a number of conditions that can endanger both the foetus and themselves. Some of these conditions are:

High Blood Pressure

Women who normally don't have high blood pressure often develop elevated readings during the second 20 weeks of pregnancy. Those whose readings exceed 140/90 must be monitored throughout the full term of their pregnancies. Hypertensive women should follow a low salt diet, monitor their weight gain and may have to take blood pressure medication.

Pre-eclampsia

Some women will accumulate excessive tissue fluid and their hands, face and legs will swell. If women who retain fluid also have protein in their urine, it means that they have pre-eclampsia. This condition can cause frontal headaches, blurred vision, upper right abdominal pain and overactive reflexes. If untreated, pre-eclampsia can turn into *eclampsia,* an emergency characterized by convulsions that violently shake the entire body, causing loss of consciousness and endangering both mother and foetus.

Blood Clots

Pregnant women may develop clots in the deep veins of their legs. Clots are formed because the pregnant uterus slows the return of blood through the leg veins and because chemicals that promote clotting increase. Clots may break free and travel to the lungs (pulmonary emboli), an emergency that can be fatal.

Vaginal Bleeding

In the first 20 weeks of pregnancy, bleeding usually indicates spontaneous termination of pregnancy, which may be accompanied by pain, cramping, tenderness and fever.

Placenta Praevia and Placental Abruption

Bleeding in the second 20 weeks is usually due to placenta praevia or placental abruption.

Placenta praevia occurs when the developing foetus pushes an abnormally low-lying placenta off the uterine wall, causing severe shock, fainting, paleness and an extremely weak pulse. Patients develop bright red bleeding that may be painless. At first, bleeding is slight, but it recurs and worsens over several days.

Placental abruption occurs when the placenta prematurely separates from its normal location on the upper uterine wall. Usually, it entails profuse, dark and often clotted vaginal bleeding, which causes severe shock, fainting, paleness and an extremely weak pulse. However, blood can be trapped between the placenta and the uterine wall, giving no obvious signs of bleeding. Women may report abdominal, pelvic or back pain. High blood pressure and physical trauma may also result in placental abruption.

Cancer, Polyps, Kidney Infections and Other Conditions

All of these conditions can cause vaginal bleeding and threaten the foetus.

What to Look for

- Fluid retention and swollen hands, face and legs throughout the day (*pre-eclampsia*).
- Frontal headaches, blurred vision, upper right abdominal pain and overactive reflexes (*pre-eclampsia*).

- Uncontrollable shaking throughout the body, followed by stiffness, confusion and disorientation (*eclampsia*).
- Pain, swelling and warmth in either calf (*deep-vein thrombosis*).
- Vaginal bleeding with cramping, tenderness or fever in the first 20 weeks of pregnancy (*spontaneous termination of pregnancy*).
- Paleness, cold and clammy skin and agitation (*excessive blood loss*).
- Painless, bright red vaginal bleeding in the second 20 weeks of pregnancy (*placenta praevia*).
- Vaginal bleeding that is heavy, dark and clotted. Shock, fainting, paleness and an extremely weak pulse in the second 20 weeks of pregnancy (*placental abruption*).
- Uterine contractions and gush of fluid before the expected date of delivery (*premature rupture of membranes*).
- Abdominal pain is not common in pregnancy and may indicate a potential emergency.
- Nausea and vomiting are common, especially in the morning (morning sickness) but should still be checked out with your doctor.

What to Do

- If a pregnant woman begins to shake uncontrollably over her entire body and then becomes stiff, confused and disoriented, call 999 immediately. You should assume that the patient has eclampsia if she has such seizures in the second half of pregnancy.
- Patients with swelling, pain and warmness in either calf may have a blood clot. Call 999 at once and keep them sitting or lying down.
- When patients bleed vaginally and have cramps, tenderness, fever, paleness, coldness, clammy skin or agitation (spontaneous termination of pregnancy, placental injury), call 999 immediately.

What Not to Do

- Don't let patients with leg pain stand, walk, or be active. They may have blood clots in their legs that could dislodge, travel to the lungs and impair the circulation of oxygen to vital organs.

Typical Treatment

The first step in treating obstetric emergencies is to check and stabilize the patient's circulation and blood flow. An ultrasound scan will then determine the age and the condition of the foetus. Lab tests will reveal the extent of blood loss and the approximate duration of the pregnancy.

Pre-eclampsia

Patients with blood pressure over 140/90 and those with lower readings who exhibit any suspicious signs or symptoms, will be hospitalized. Pre-eclampsia requires bed rest, blood pressure monitoring and frequent visits by the obstetrician. Seizures affecting eclampsia patients will be controlled with intravenous magnesium sulfate or antiepileptic and blood pressure medication. When the patient's condition has stabilized, a decision will be made whether to deliver the child by Caesarean section or allow the pregnancy to continue. It may be safer to care for a premature newborn in the neonatal intensive care unit than to let it remain in the mother's uterus where it could be injured if the mother has convulsions or circulatory problems. Eclampsia is thought to be triggered by the release of hormones during pregnancy and usually resolves after delivery.

Phlebitis

Patients with blood clots will be hospitalized and given intravenous blood thinners. Specialized radiological testing such as Doppler ultrasound scans and venography will show whether clots have dissolved and normal blood flow has been restored. If there is risk of haemorrhage or the mother's death, a decision must be made at the thirty-fourth to thirty-sixth week of gestation whether or not to deliver the baby (and transfer it to a neonatal intensive care unit).

Placental Injury
Placental abruption and bleeding placenta praevia patients will immediately receive intravenous fluids and oxygen. They may be rushed to the delivery room for Caesarean delivery. Newborns are then monitored in the intensive care unit and the mothers will remain hospitalized until their conditions stabilize.

Premature Labour/Rupture of Membranes
New medications (tocolytics) can inhibit labour contractions for several days and provide time for the mother to get to a facility with a neonatal ICU. Among the drugs available are terbutaline, magnesium sulfate, nifedipine and corticosteroids. They may be used only if the foetus is between 24 to 34 weeks of gestation.

After-care
Obstetric emergencies are extremely serious and often require a week or more of postnatal hospitalization. Massive bleeding and pelvic infections are two emergencies that commonly occur during the postnatal period, requiring observation in the hospital for several days after delivery.

Doctor Says

Monitor all pregnancies whether they are high-risk or not to reduce the risk of unhappy complications. Remember – obstetric problems involve both the lives of expectant mothers and their children. Since many of the same problems can recur during subsequent pregnancies, mothers should get frequent check-ups to monitor their condition if they become pregnant again.

Procedures

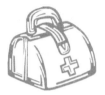

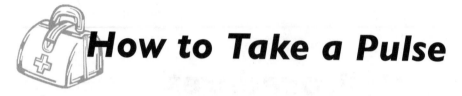

How to Take a Pulse

Our heart pumps blood through the body in a regular rhythm or cadence. At certain points on the body, we can feel that rhythm or pulse and measure its beat. If we feel a pulse, we know that the heart is beating, which means that the patient is alive. If we count the number of beats, we can calculate the rate or strength with which the heart is beating.

Although the pulse can be felt at a number of locations, the easiest places for most people to access are the wrist and carotid artery in the neck. Finding a pulse can be frustrating, especially the first few times you try. So practise on yourself and/or on your family so you can find a pulse quickly in a medical emergency.

In medical emergencies, don't bother to calculate the patient's pulse rate. Simply try to find the patient's pulse and estimate whether it is beating strongly, weakly, or not at all. If the patient isn't breathing and you can't find a pulse within ten seconds, begin CPR.

To take a pulse:

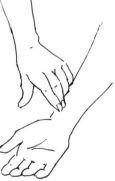

On the Wrist
Place the pads of your index and middle fingers on the groove on the inner side of the patient's wrist just up the arm from the bone at the base of the thumb (about 2cm/1in up from the place where the hand meets the wrist). Move your fingers lightly until you feel intermittent pulsations.

How to Take a Pulse

On the Neck
Lift the chin slightly and lightly run the pads of your three middle fingers along the outer edge of the windpipe under the patient's jaw and alongside the Adam's apple. Keep moving your fingers until you feel an intermittent throb – the pulse.

Calculating the Pulse Rate
Once you have found the pulse, press gently and keep your fingers in place. Then count the number of pulse beats you feel in a ten-second period. Multiply the number of pulse beats by six to get the patient's pulse rate per minute.

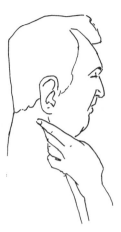

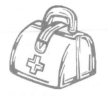

How to Give CPR

Cardiopulmonary resuscitation (CPR) is used to try to revive patients who are not breathing and/or have no heartbeat (pulse). It is used when patients have:

- Collapsed and are unresponsive.
- Stopped breathing.
- No pulse.
- Blue lips, fingers or face.

What to Do

1. Check the patient's responsiveness:
   - Gently tap the patient's shoulder and ask, 'Are you okay?' Speak loudly and repeat several times, if necessary. Patients who have had a heart attack, or serious head injury, or taken a drug overdose, may not respond, but those who are simply intoxicated, have fainted or are asleep will usually answer promptly.
   - Check the patient's breathing. Remove or open clothing to see if the chest rises and falls. Place your ear by the nose and mouth to hear or feel the passage of air. If, after several seconds, there is no chest movement, proceed as if the patient is unresponsive.

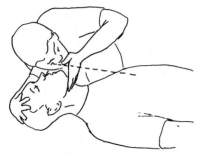

2. Call 999, even if you have to leave the patient alone. If you are not alone, someone should stay with the patient while another person calls 999. Time is of the essence: the sooner trained emergency medical personnel arrive and begin advanced cardiac life support, the greater the chances of survival.

3. Immediately place the patient flat on his/her back and elevate the legs slightly to improve circulation to the vital organs. However, *don't move patients with suspected neck injuries*!

4. Tilt the head back slightly to establish an airway. If necessary, place your hand under the patient's neck to lift his/her chin upward and forward to fully open the mouth. This will also prevent the tongue from blocking airflow to and from the lungs.

5. Administer *mouth-to-mouth ventilation*:

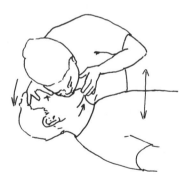

   - Take a deep breath.
   - Pinch the patient's nostrils.
   - Place your mouth directly on the patient's mouth.
   - Slowly exhale fully into the patient's mouth filling up his/her lungs.
   - Repeat one more time.
   - Check that the patient's chest rises and falls between breaths (to see that the air goes in).
   - If the lungs fail to expand, the patient may have an upper airway obstruction. If so, see page 198.
   - Observe the patient's chest and put your ear to the mouth and nose to determine if the victim is breathing on his/her own.

6. Place two fingers (other than your thumb) on the (carotid) artery that runs to the side of the Adam's apple and feel for a pulse. If you find a pulse, some functions (breathing and heart) may have been restored, but the patient's blood pressure and normal circulation may still be impaired.

7. If you don't feel a pulse after ten seconds, immediately begin chest compressions. Kneel next to the patient with your knees by the victim's shoulder and upper arm.

For Adults

Place the heel of one hand 5cm (2in) above the centre of the lower tip of the patient's breastbone and the other hand directly on top of it, so that one hand covers most of the other. Move your torso directly over the patient so your arms point straight down towards his chest. With your elbows straight and locked, press directly down on the breastbone 4–5cm (1½–2in). Apply pressure with the heel of your lower palm, not with your fingers, which could fracture a rib. Hold each compression for about one second.

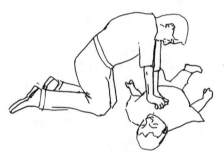

For Children

• Press with the heel of *one* hand only to compress the breastbone about 2cm (1in).
• Place the other hand on the forehead to keep the airway open.

How to Give CPR

For Infants

- Use two fingers of one hand to compress the breastbone about 1cm (1/2in)
- Continue CPR without stopping until emergency help arrives.

One-Rescuer CPR

- If alone, compress the chest 15 times.
- Give two (2) mouth-to-mouth ventilations.
- Continue the 15-to-2 ratio until emergency medical personnel arrive.
- Periodically check to see if the patient's heart has begun to beat (feel the neck/carotid artery) or there is spontaneous breathing. After a few seconds, if there is neither breathing nor a heartbeat, resume CPR.

Two-Rescuer CPR

- One person should apply chest compressions while the other gives mouth-to-mouth ventilation.
- Give five (5) chest compressions followed immediately by one (1) mouth-to-mouth ventilation.
- Continue this 5-to-1 pattern until emergency medical personnel arrive.
- To avoid fatigue, rescuers should rotate duties and, in the interval when they switch, check if the patient is breathing or has a heartbeat.
- If the patient begins breathing and his/her heart begins beating, place the patient on his/her side.

What Not to Do

- Don't move patients who may have neck injuries.
- In giving chest compressions, don't apply pressure with your fingers because the force could break a rib. Instead, press straight downward with the heel of your hand.

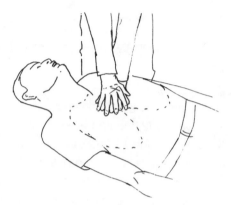

Typical Treatment

When emergency medical personnel arrive, they will continue CPR. They'll also give advanced cardiac life support – treatment that improves oxygenation, treats potentially lethal heart rhythm disturbances and may restore blood pressure and circulation.

Survivors of heart attack will be hospitalized and monitored in an intensive care unit. Dangerous heart rhythms often occur during the first 24 hours; these may require immediate administration of intravenous medication or electrical defibrillation. The length of a patient's hospitalization will depend on the gravity of each individual case.

Doctor Says

When you call 999, help won't arrive for several minutes at least, so your ability to perform CPR may keep the patient alive. Learn CPR. The St John Ambulance, St Andrew's Ambulance Association and the British Red Cross all offer courses on first aid, including the skills needed to perform this often life-saving therapy.

There is no evidence of HIV being contracted through mouth-to-mouth ventilation. Experts believe that saliva protects first-aiders, so CPR should never be delayed to look for plastic shields, tissues or other forms of protection. Emergency medical personnel use specialized ventilation equipment.

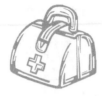

How to Dislodge an Obstruction from the Throat

What to Look for

- Coughing, gasping for air and/or clutching the throat.
- Fast and deep breathing.
- Change in patient's voice (partial obstruction)/inability to talk (total obstruction).
- Wheezing (from trying to force air around the trapped object).
- Blue fingers, lips and face.
- Collapse, unconsciousness.

What to Do

Conscious Patients

- Keep patients erect, with their heads leaning slightly forward. Call 999 immediately if they can talk, cough and breathe without assistance. Allow alert patients with partial obstruction to try to clear the blockage on their own.
- If the patient can't talk, breathe or cough, bend their head forward until it is lower than their chest and give five (5) blows between shoulder blades, using the flat of the hand. Place a

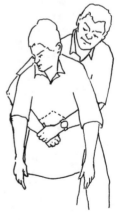

198

child over your knee and slap him/her between the shoulder blades, using less force than for an adult. Place an infant along your forearm and slap using even less force.

- If this fails to clear the obstruction, perform five (5) abdominal thrusts (Heimlich manoeuvre). Only perform on adults, and children over the age of one year old.

  1. Stand directly behind the patient.
  2. Wrap your arms around the patient's waist.
  3. Clasp your hands above the navel, under the ribcage, so your thumb is pressing against the patient's abdomen. Be sure your hands are several inches below the lower tip of the patient's breastbone.
  4. Pull inward and upward five (5) times in succession.
  5. After each cycle of five (5) thrusts, gently sweep the patient's mouth with your finger to see if the object has popped out and can be removed.
  6. Repeat the cycle of five (5) abdominal thrusts until the object dislodges, the person becomes unconscious or collapses, or emergency personnel arrive.

Infants under one year old

Place the infant on your lap, face up. Place two (2) fingers between the navel and ribcage and compress downward and towards the shoulders several times.

Unconscious Patients

- Call 999 immediately.
- If a patient inhaled vomit, turn the victim onto his/her side with the head back. This should move the tongue forward and allow gastric contents to empty out of the mouth, not into the lungs.

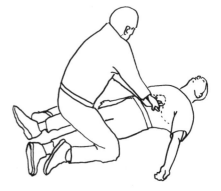

How to Dislodge an Obstruction from the Throat

1. Turn the patient on his/her back and kneel along side his/her hips facing their head.
2. Deliver five (5) abdominal thrusts (Heimlich manoeuvre) by:
   a. Pressing the heels of your hands above the patient's navel, several inches under the ribcage. Be sure your hands are below the lower tip of the breastbone.
   b. Push inward towards the shoulders five (5) times in succession.
   c. After each cycle, gently sweep the patient's mouth with your finger to see if the object has popped out and can be removed.
   d. Repeating the cycle of five (5) abdominal thrusts and checking the patient's mouth until the obstructing object is dislodged, the person becomes conscious, or emergency personnel arrive.

Choking Infants
- Place the child on his/her back.
- Place two (2) fingers between the navel and ribcage and compress downward and towards the shoulders several times.
- Check the child's mouth to see if the object has popped out and can be removed. Proceed cautiously because it is easy to push objects back into the windpipe. Continue until help arrives.

If You Are Choking
- Stand facing the back of a chair or over a railing.
- Place your fist between your navel and ribcage.
- Lean downward quickly into the chair or railing so that your fist presses into the abdomen and upward towards the shoulders.
- Repeat until the object pops out, you can breathe normally or help arrives.

How to Stop Bleeding Wounds

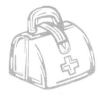

Most bleeding from wounds can be stopped when you apply pressure directly on the wound. Otherwise you may be able to apply pressure to a major artery – use this only when direct pressure fails, and for not more than ten minutes.

What to Do

- Call 999 immediately.
- Remove or cut the patient's clothing to find the wound.
- Press directly on the wound. If possible use a clean dressing, absorbent pads, bandages, gauze or cloth.
- If the bleeding is severe and no clean dressings are readily available, use your fingers or the palm of your hand. (Don't spend too long looking for clean dressings if loss of blood may put the patient's life at risk.)
- Maintain pressure until the bleeding stops.
- Do not remove the dressing even after it becomes saturated with blood. If necessary, place other dressings over the saturated ones.
- For injuries to limbs, lift the wounded arm or leg until it is above heart level. Don't elevate a broken limb.
- If direct pressure to an arm or leg wound does not stop the bleeding, try to find the pressure point with the hand that is not applying direct pressure on the wound and apply pressure on the pressure point.

- Feel for the pulse on the inner side of the upper arm (brachial artery) or top of the leg near the groin (femoral artery) and apply pressure there. Do this for no longer than 10 minutes.

How to Support Fractures

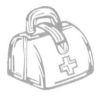

If you suspect a fracture, the first priority is to immobilize the break. Support the injury above and below, padding with pillows, towels or cushions, to make the patient comfortable. An arm fracture, if the patient can bend the limb, may be secured with a sling (see page 205) or bandages, or you can use a safety pin to attach the patient's sleeve to a shirt, blouse or other garment. If the patient is mobile, transport them to A&E. Otherwise phone 999. Always phone 999 for serious injuries, especially if the bone protrudes through the flesh (open fracture) or the injury involves the head, neck or back.

In most parts of the UK, emergency personnel will soon arrive to deal with serious injuries, so your main priorities are to stay with the patient, keep them calm, discourage them from moving and keep them as comfortable as possible. You may need to place your hands above and below the wound, or use padding to support the limb until help arrives. If medical help may be delayed (in remote areas, say) you can immobilize broken or dislocated bones, sprains and strains with bandages and splints. For example, you may be able to immobilize a leg fracture by using bandages to secure the broken limb to the uninjured one.

Immobilizing injuries prevents fractured bones from moving and so prevents further injury, reduces pain and limits shock. Any rigid item can be used as a splint, if it is long enough to secure the fracture and the joints above and below. You can improvize with a broom, umbrella, stick, board, pipe – even tightly rolled newspaper.

How to Make Splints

What to Do

- Loosen or remove tight or constricting clothing. Remove jewellery that could cut off circulation when the injured area swells. Put the jewellery in the patient's pocket.
- Try not to move injured limbs. If this is impossible, gently lift the injured limb with both hands in one motion without disturbing any broken bones – get others to help, if possible. Then carefully position the injured limb as below.
- For an arm fracture, if the patient cannot bend the limb, help them lie down. Place the broken arm alongside the body, put padding between the arm and the body and secure in place using bandages, scarves, cut-up clothing (or other suitable material).
- For a leg fracture, place a long splint between the legs Cushion the splint with soft padding, such as blankets, towels or clothing, especially where a splint touches an ankle or other bony area. Secure with bandages rope, belt, ties, scarves, fabric strips (or other suitable material). Secure ankles and knees together first, then immobilize above and below the fracture. For a thigh fracture, you may need to secure another, longer splint on the outside of the limb – from armpit to ankle.
- Bandages or other ties should be firm enough to prevent movement – but don't cut off circulation and try not to wrap or knot the fastenings directly over the site of the injury. You may need to retie if the limb swells.
- Once splints are secure, elevate the limb above heart level to minimize swelling.
- Regularly check the circulation in the injured limb. Check for painful swelling, blue or pale skin, cold, pins and needles or numbing, and loosen fastenings if necessary.

What Not to Do

- Don't move a patient if you even remotely suspect a broken neck.
- Don't try to align or set a broken bone.

How to Make Slings

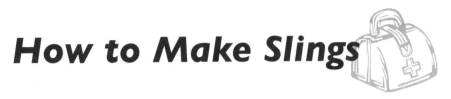

Essentially, a sling is a bandage draped around a patient's neck to immobilize, support and protect an injured arm from further damage. Triangular cloths, bandages or scarves make ideal slings, but if unavailable you can improvise by using and often cutting up, clothing and other nonstretch material (even tights can be used).

What to Do

1. Use a triangular cloth, bandage or any nonstretch material that can be tied around the patient's neck to hold the injured arm (such as a tie, belt or pieces of clothing).

2. Put one corner of the triangle around the patient's neck on the side opposite to the injury. Then place another corner so that it is pointing downward and the third by the patient's elbow.

3. Gently bend the injured arm so that the patient's hand is slightly higher than his/her elbow and across his/her chest.

4. Place the injured arm in the broadest part of the triangle and adjust it so that the support does not press directly on the injured area.

5. Tie the corner around the patient's neck with the corner that originally pointed downward so that the patient's arm is cushioned at slightly less than a 90° angle (hand higher than elbow).

How to Make Slings

6. Tie the sling with a knot at the side of the patient's neck opposite the injury and cushion the knot with cloth or a handkerchief so that it doesn't dig into the patient.

7. Secure the patient's injured arm to his/her torso by wrapping a bandage, rope, or fabric over the injured arm, around the back and under the uninjured arm.

Measuring Vital Signs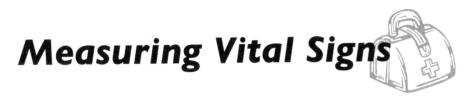

Measuring a patient's vital signs provides invaluable information on the patient's condition. In medical emergencies, ambulance personnel, paramedics and A&E doctors and nurses will check a patient's vital signs while they ask some basic questions, before they begin any tests or treatments. The vital signs will help them determine the nature of the patient's problem. The vital signs that are measured are:

- Temperature.
- Heart rate.
- Breathing rate.
- Blood pressure.

Any disorder that depletes the body of water, tissue fluid or blood will lower blood pressure and trigger an accelerated heart rate. When body temperature is raised by just one degree, the pulse increases by ten beats per minute.

Blood circulates oxygen throughout the body and must be chemically balanced for us to function properly. Diseases that increase the amount of dissolved acid in the blood produce a state of acidosis (kidney failure, asthma) and cause the patient's respiratory rate to rise (over the normal 18 breaths per minute). Illnesses that slow the heart (certain rhythm disturbances) or breathing (opiate overdoses) can abruptly change the pH (acid-alkaline) balance of the blood and tissues and stop the heart.

Shock

Patients go 'into shock' when their blood circulation becomes critically poor and jeopardizes vital organs. When cells in the heart, brain and kidneys are deprived of oxygen for several minutes they die. Patients in shock usually have very low blood pressure, often under 80/50. Shock can be brought on by severe fluid and/or blood loss from burns or an injured artery, by impaired pumping of blood during a heart attack, as well as by blood-borne infections, severe allergic reactions and spinal cord injuries.

Mental Status

In the A&E unit, the staff will usually check a 'fifth vital sign': the patient's mental status. Many medical emergencies can change a patient's levels of orientation, awareness and thinking. Reflexes can dramatically change and the patient may be unable to move or communicate. A wide variety of conditions can alter a patient's mental status including injury (bleeding into the brain), infections (encephalitis, meningitis) and intoxication from alcohol and/or drugs. Examples of heightened forms of altered mental status are agitation, delirium and dementia. Stupor and coma are states of depressed or absent brain activity. A patient's mental status may change during the course of his/her observation (for better or worse), which may provide information that will help in diagnosing the source of the problem.

Emergency Supply Kits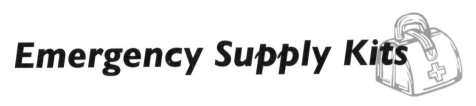

Create an emergency supply kit for your home, place of business, vehicle or boat. Use the list below as a guideline to stock a kit that meets your needs. In creating a kit, consider factors such as where you live and your distance from an emergency care centre (especially on holiday or if living in remote, rural areas). Also factor in who might need first aid care and whether they suffer from any particular medical conditions.

You probably have many of the items listed below already, so just fill in the gaps because you never know when you may need them. Check the expiry dates on all your supplies. Many first aid supplies should be replaced after one year.

A number of vendors sell prepackaged, emergency supply kits, including the St John Ambulance, the St Andrew's Ambulance Association and the British Red Cross. Many come in durable, weatherproof containers.

Supply Kit Checklist

- A copy of this book
- Disposable protective gloves
- Torch and extra batteries
- EpiPen® (for adrenaline injection)
- Sharp knife
- Scissors and/or shears
- Tweezers
- Thermometer
- Blankets
- Water: 5.5 litres (8 pints) per person per day for 3 days
- Plastic bags, assorted sizes

- Waterproof adhesive tape (duct tape)
- Waterproof adhesive dressings and plasters, in assorted sizes
- Hypoallergenic adhesive dressings and plasters, in assorted sizes
- Triangular bandages
- Tubular bandages (for injuries to fingers and joints)
- Crêpe roller bandages
- Butterfly closures (to secure bandages and dressings)
- Safety pins, medium size
- Sterile cotton wool
- Gauze pads in assorted sizes
- Gauze rolls
- Sanitary napkins
- Tissues
- Alcohol cleansing pads
- Antiseptic wipes
- Absorbent lint
- Cotton wool swabs

- Instant-activating cold packs
- Instant-activating heat packs
- Aspirin and/or ibuprofen (for general pain relief and inflammatory joint pain)
- Paracetamol (for general pain relief and to reduce high temperature)
- Children's paracetamol (e.g. Calpol)
- Antacid
- Travel sickness pills
- Antidiarrhoeal medicine
- Antihistamine/anti-allergy pills (for sting or food allergies)
- Decongestant tablets or nasal spray
- Calamine lotion
- Antiseptic lotion or ointment
- Anti-itching ointment
- Burn relief gel packs
- Sunblock
- Survival bags (to keep casualties warm)
- Plastic face shield (for protection when giving mouth-to-mouth ventilation)

Tips for Travellers

How To Prepare For Medical Emergencies When You Are Away From Home

Whether you are out jogging near your home or travelling in a foreign country, it is a good idea to carry a card that has vital information about your health. This card should contain the following information, but you may want to add to it:

1. Your name and the address and the phone number where you are staying.

2. Name of a person to contact in an emergency.

3. Any medical problems or allergies you may have, including allergy to medication.

4. List of medications you are taking.

5. Your doctor's name, address and phone number.

If you have a mobile phone, carry it with you. It could be your lifeline in an emergency.

If you have a potentially serious health problem and are staying at a hotel or someone's home, ask where the nearest hospital is. Find out what the procedure is to get you there if the need arises.

For Travel Abroad

1. Before you leave, find out what vaccinations you need (see Travellers' Web Sites, page 214), and check up on any current disease outbreaks in areas where you plan to travel.

2. Schedule vaccinations well in advance. Get your injections early because they may take time to take effect and certain countries will bar your entry if your immunization is not yet effective. In addition, some vaccinations may entail a series of inoculations and you may have adverse reactions that could delay the process. Finally, GPs are not equipped to give all the immunizations you may need so you may have to go to a special travel health centre, which could take time to locate, schedule and visit.

3. See your GP for a physical examination, to get all necessary booster injections and to update your prescriptions. Get a written copy of all your prescriptions and have your doctor write down their generic names so that they can be easily understood and filled abroad.

4. Have your doctor complete a personal medical record for you to carry during your travels. The record should list your chronic medical conditions, recent disorders, allergies and blood type. Also carry your doctor's name, address and phone number.

5. Carry your prescription medicines in their original containers with their original labels or carry copies of your prescriptions signed by your doctor. This can facilitate getting refills and avoid hassles with customs officials.

6. If you have private health insurance, check to see if it covers the treatment of medical emergencies abroad.

7. If your private health insurance doesn't cover medical emergencies abroad, purchase a supplemental travel health insurance policy or an emergency assistance policy through your travel agent or insurance agent. Make sure that the policy covers medical evacuation, which can be enormously expensive. Most companies that cover medical emergencies abroad provide 24-hour phone support and will direct you to doctors and hospitals. Some will send cheques to pay your emergency medical costs, which can be important since many foreign medical providers won't invoice your insurance carrier and insist on payment on the spot.

8. Leave a copy of your itinerary with a reliable friend or member of your family. Include in your itinerary all your air, sea and ground travel departure and arrival times; all flight, ship and train numbers; the name, address and phone number of your hotels or places where you will be staying and your doctor's name and phone number.

9. Should you incur any medical problems abroad, make an appointment upon your return to see and discuss it with your doctor or an appropriate specialist. Parasites and exposures to exotic illnesses are an inherent risk of foreign travel. In addition, aeroplanes are enclosed compartments that act as incubators for airborne illness.

10. Pack an emergency supply kit (see page 209) that is appropriate for the countries you will be visiting and the types of activity you are planning. Remember, the more adventurous the holiday, the more comprehensive the kit. (Consider including disposable syringes and hypodermic needles if you are planning to visit countries where hygiene standards – especially hepatitis and HIV risk – may be open to doubt.)

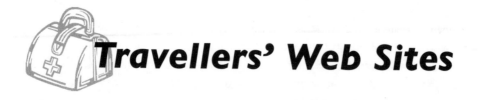

Travellers' Web Sites

UK citizens undertake up to 60 million foreign trips every year. Yet surveys show that less than two-thirds of travellers to areas of moderate-to-high disease risk seek medical advice before setting off, and over half do not get all the required vaccinations. Even some of the most popular holiday destinations in Europe and North America carry serious health risks, including life-threatening infectious diseases. The following web sites provide vital information for all travellers on foreign medical care, important vaccinations and other measures to prevent disease.

Department of Health: This UK Government web site contains advice on how to stay healthy abroad or medical get treatment if you fall ill. It includes information on the E111 UK Citizen's Passport to free/reduced-cost emergency care in most European countries. The Department of Health also publishes the 'Yellow Book' – *Health Information for Overseas Travel* (HMSO).

www.dh.gov.uk/PolicyAndGuidance/HealthAdviceforTravellers/fs/en

World Health Organization (WHO): The WHO's international web site has all the latest information on current disease threats through its worldwide system of monitoring, mapping and surveillance. You can also download advice on:
– Accidents, injuries and violence
– Blood transfusions

- Countries endemic for yellow fever
- Country list: vaccination requirements
- Environmental health risks
- Health risks and precautions – general considerations
- Infectious diseases of potential risk to travellers
- International health regulations
- Malaria situation
- Travel by air – health considerations
- Vaccine preventable diseases, vaccines and vaccinations

www.who.int/ith/en/

Centers for Disease Control and Prevention (CDC): A US Government web site that features a wide range of health advice for travellers. Although mainly intended for US citizens, for travellers from the UK it is particularly useful for advice on travel in South and Central America.

www.cdc.gov/travel/

Fit for Travel: This web site, provided by the NHS (Scotland), gives a broad range of travel health information for all UK citizens, including advice for special needs travellers, parents travelling with children, vaccinations, disease risks, and practical travel tips compiled by British Embassies. Customised travel information is also available by post.

www.fitfortravel.scot.nhs.uk/Home.html

Medical Advisory Service for Travellers Abroad (MASTA): Run in conjunction with the London School of Hygiene and Tropical Medicine, this web site gives information on travel health and vaccinations, including advice on preventing mosquito-borne diseases such as malaria and yellow fever, and how to find your nearest travel clinic.

www.masta.org/

Foreign & Commonwealth Office: Up-to-date advice and information on current global dangers when travelling abroad, including disease, environmental risks, civil disorder, terrorism and crime.

www.fco.gov.uk

UK Vaccine Industry Group (UVIG): Information, including fact sheets, on vaccines and vaccine-preventable diseases.

www.uvig.org/faqsheets/travel.asp

Travelhealth Disease Prevention: Information on diseases, NHS and WHO vaccination recommendations, disease maps, travel clinics and a vaccination chart to help you keep your vaccinations up to day and remind you of booster injections.

www.travelhealth.co.uk/diseases/

Malaria Hotspots: Information on malaria and its prevention, including high-risk zones, plus general travel advice.

www.malariahotspots.co.uk

National Travel Health Network and Centre (NaTHNaC): Advice for GP practices and other health care providers on travel health topics, including current disease epidemics, insect bite prevention, food and water hygiene and sun care.

www.nathnac.org/travel/index.htm

British Airways – Health and Well Being: Health and medical advice for air travellers, including wheelchair users and others requiring special assistance.

www.britishairways.com/travel/health

Index

Index

Index

THE BOOK OF
MEDICAL
EMERGENCIES